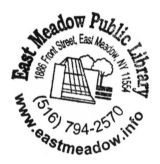

FATAL

CONVENIENCES

ALSO BY DARIN OLIEN

SuperLife: The 5 Simple Fixes That Will Make
You Healthy, Fit, and Eternally Awesome

FATAL
CONVENIENCES

The Toxic Products and Harmful Habits
That Are Making You Sick—and the Simple
Changes That Will Save Your Health

DARIN OLIEN

HARPER WAVE

An Imprint of HarperCollins*Publishers*

FATAL CONVENIENCES. Copyright © 2023 by Darin Olien. All rights reserved. Printed in the United States of America. No part of this book may be used or reproduced in any manner whatsoever without written permission except in the case of brief quotations embodied in critical articles and reviews. For information, address HarperCollins Publishers, 195 Broadway, New York, NY 10007.

HarperCollins books may be purchased for educational, business, or sales promotional use. For information, please email the Special Markets Department at SPsales@harpercollins.com.

FIRST EDITION

Designed by Nancy Singer

Library of Congress Cataloging-in-Publication Data has been applied for.

ISBN 978-0-06-311453-1

23 24 25 26 27 LBC 5 4 3 2 1

I dedicate this book to my late father, Howard Olien. He suffered from chemical sensitivities long before people knew such a thing even existed. Now I am passing the lessons he taught me on to you in the hope that no one else will have to suffer.

CONTENTS

5 FOOD AND BEVERAGES

When you realize that many of the things we consume in order to stay alive contain harmful substances that can make us ill, it's a little depressing. But the truth is that the easier something is to eat and drink, the worse it is for our health.

6 ELECTROMAGNETIC RADIATION

You can't see it, hear it, or smell it, and it emanates from the coolest things we own: our electronic tools and toys. By now, they all feel more like necessities than conveniences. No wonder we'd rather not think about the invisible hazards of the tech we love.

7 CLOTHING

With all the obvious dangers that surround us, we might never suspect that our clothes might also be hurting us. Well, guess again! Even our apparel contains quite a few conveniences, and some of those are not doing us any favors.

8 HOUSEHOLD PRODUCTS

We love our homes and do our best to make them friendly, welcoming, and clean. So how can it be that the safest, most comfortable place in the world is filled with so many hazardous, toxic, and sketchy bad influences?

9 SOME FINAL THOUGHTS

Just a few parting words before I let you go.

10 OKAY, SO *NOW* WHAT SHOULD WE DO?

Believe it or not, there's good news amid all these Fatal Conveniences: Today, there are many nonfatal alternatives that make life easy and enjoyable without making us sick and killing us or the planet. Here I provide a ton of good sources and even some DIY solutions.

ACKNOWLEDGMENTS

It takes a village to write a book, especially this one. Here's where I give many, many thanks.

FATAL

CONVENIENCES

INTRODUCTION

I LOVE CONVENIENCES.

We all do! And for good reason—they make our lives so much better. Easier. Without conveniences, life would be really hard. It would suck.

Here's an example of a pretty amazing convenience we all enjoy: the wheel! Try to picture what life would be like if someone hadn't come up with the wheel way back whenever. Hard to imagine. But definitely a drag.

Here's another great one: fire! Think of all the awesome things that happened once we managed to create and control fire and heat. We wouldn't recognize our lives without it. It goes way beyond just making things easier.

I could spend all day naming wonderful conveniences: The internal combustion engine. Electrical power. Indoor plumbing. Flight. Agriculture. Wi-Fi. True, we could live without them. But life wouldn't be as much fun.

This book is a convenience. Somebody—a team of us, actually—had to research a long list of subjects and then organize the information and explain what it means and package it in a form that you could understand and easily use. What if everybody interested in this subject had to spend days and weeks wading through scientific literature, trying to make sense of it, and then come up with advice on the best way to live? Not many people would do all that on their own.

But we don't have to—thanks to our gift for conveniences.

I was about to say it's human nature to find ways of making life easier and more efficient. But the truth is that *all* animals love conveniences. I just read about some cockatoos in Australia that figured out how to open garbage cans so they could eat what was inside. Some birds taught themselves the skill, while others watched until they learned to do it, too. Still other cockatoos just waited until everybody else finished eating, at which point they fed on the leftovers—a lot less work than scrounging for dinner old school.

I live with two German shepherds, a six-year-old named Chaga and a four-year-old named Ella. They wouldn't even exist if ten thousand or so years ago some wolves hadn't discovered that if they hung around humans, they could eat their food scraps, which was a hell of a lot easier than chasing down prey and killing it.

So it's obvious that all living creatures love conveniences and are excellent at inventing them. It's like a force of nature. It's who we are. It's a great thing.

Until, of course . . .

Until we go too far, and the conveniences we create start making us sick and killing us. Then they're not so great. They're not so great once they start causing cancers and other terrible diseases or when they disrupt our ability to make babies or when they trash our environment and hurt every living thing and the planet itself. Then conveniences aren't so cool.

That's what I'm going to talk about in this book—the Fatal Conveniences that claim to help us but instead do us harm—even cause death, believe it or not.

But don't worry, my mission is *not* to make your life more inconvenient or to scare you away from using the conveniences you love. It's to expose the ones that are damaging us, and show that it's possible to find terrific products that are *not* fatal and are *not* harmful to ourselves and our world. That's our goal. And I have some amazing, wonderful things to show you along the way.

Let's get going!

1

WHAT IS A FATAL CONVENIENCE?

LET'S START WITH A PARTIAL LIST, just so you know what's in store.

Personal care products, like:

Soap and bodywash

Shampoo

Fragrance

Moisturizer and skin lotion

Antiaging creams

Petroleum jelly

Cosmetics

Tampons

Shaving cream

Sunscreen

Deodorant

Toothpaste

Mouthwash

Household items, including:

Laundry detergent

Dryer sheets

Furniture
Carpeting
Air-conditioning
Bedding
Cleaning products
Air fresheners
Cookware
Plastic containers
Aluminum foil
Plastic wrap

Electronic devices, like:

Microwave ovens
Modems and Wi-Fi
Computers and tablets
Cell phones
Bluetooth headphones

Food and drink, including:

Snack foods
Nonorganic produce
Conventionally raised meat and poultry
Nutritional supplements
Energy drinks
Dairy products
Bottled water and other beverages

And some random things you might never suspect, such as:

Jeans
Dental floss
Dry cleaning chemicals
Diapers

Fast-food wrappers
T-shirts

This includes a lot of stuff we all use every day, right?

The list of Fatal Conveniences is almost endless, and it constantly grows longer as new products and novel substances are introduced into the marketplace and our homes and lives. There are so many more, but this is a good start on the major ones.

Over the past fifty or so years, more than 80,000 chemicals have been introduced into our environment, and the vast majority weren't tested first to see if they were safe for human contact. We know for a fact that at least 1,500 of them are suspected of being carcinogenic. Many times—more often than not—we don't even know that these substances are contained in the things we use every day.

How insane is that? We're buying them, eating them, putting them onto our skin, bringing them into our homes, but what exactly are they? Most of the time, we have no idea!

In lots of cases, the damage isn't even created by the convenience itself. It's caused by a hidden, unnoticed ingredient that comes along for the ride: The preservative. The propellant. The flavoring. The dye. The emulsifier. The thickener. The lining of the container. The completely unnecessary fragrance that's there only to make you love the product a little more. The carcinogenic pesticide used in farming that's a shortcut for the big agriculture conglomerates. The sugar under an unrecognizable name. The harm that is done is often like the shadow of the thing, the aura, the invisible residue that it leaves behind. It's extra dangerous because we don't even know it's there.

Want a good example? You are probably unaware that a chemical from the same family as Teflon is used on clothing so that it won't be wrinkled after you wash it. Cool! Great idea. The only problem is that the chemical sometimes causes skin irritation, can disrupt your normal hormone function, and may even be cancer causing.

So there's the trade-off that can be found at the heart of all Fatal

Conveniences: On the one hand—no more ironing! On the other—increased risk of cancer! Worth it?

Here's another. Early in the twentieth century, scientists discovered that areas with high levels of naturally occurring fluoride in their drinking water also had low levels of tooth decay. Before long, communities across the US were adding the chemical to their tap water, and soon after, manufacturers began putting it into toothpaste. A wonderful convenience.

And then researchers learned some alarming facts about fluoride, mainly its toxic effects on the developing human brain.

"Children in high-fluoride areas had significantly lower IQ scores than those who lived in low-fluoride areas," according to one study. There were also some concerns about fluoride consumption and its relationship to bone cancer, bone fractures, and reproductive system problems.

To be fair, fluoride is a problem only if you swallow it, but try telling that to kids happily using bubble gum–flavored toothpaste. So you decide—is a mouth of cavity-free teeth worth a couple of IQ points?

Or maybe the kidney beans in that can are nutritious. But the lining of the can? Toxic. Or your new stretch jeans fit and look great. But they're shedding tiny bits of microplastic that go into your body and your environment. Wouldn't you rather get your beans and your jeans without anything gnarly on the side?

That's the kind of thing I'm going to be talking about. There's a lot to say.

I WANT TO WALK YOU through a day in the life of Fatal Conveniences.

Let's begin with something really basic but really important: how you smell. How we *all* smell. Throughout this book, as you'll see, the subject of fragrance comes up again and again. It's one of the biggest culprits in the world of Fatal Conveniences, especially when we're talking about personal care products, a very big deal in most of our lives.

We're all suckers for a pretty smell—the olfactory system is overwhelmingly powerful, the strongest of all our senses by far. You can smell something today and not again for the next couple decades, but when you're exposed to it then, you will recognize it. Can't say the same about something you saw, heard, or felt.

There's a good reason our noses are so strong: we use our olfactory sense to tell us what is safe to eat. It's why our noses are right over our mouths. In the wild, it's also good for knowing if a predator (or prey) is nearby. Smell and survival go hand in hand.

What's so bad about smelling good? Fragrance holds a special place in the world of Fatal Conveniences due to a 1966 federal law that regulates labeling and packaging of personal care products. In that law there's something known as "the fragrance loophole." It means that manufacturers don't have to list the ingredients used to give products their smell; instead they can just say "fragrance" or "parfum" on the label. That's because the way something smells is considered a trade secret, meaning that we're not allowed to know what we're putting on our bodies. As a result, your lotion, soap, or shaving cream can have any combination of the more than three thousand chemicals used to give products their aroma, and you'll never know what exactly is in a given product—or if it's hazardous to your health.

According to Janet Nudelman, co-founder of the Campaign for Safe Cosmetics, a project of the Breast Cancer Fund, "We found fragrance chemicals linked to cancer, birth defects, endocrine disruption and other serious health conditions in everything from children's shampoo to body lotion to perfumes." One chemical sometimes found in fragrance, styrene, has been labeled a human carcinogen, and others can cause allergic reactions and irritation of the skin, eyes, and lungs.

With all that in mind, let's start our day.

We wake up and shower with soap or bodywash—there's one fragrance. Shampoo, there's another. Conditioner, another. Our deodorant is a fourth, our toothpaste and mouthwash, a fifth and sixth, and if we're using skin lotion or moisturizer, we're up to seven different smells. If you're a woman who's been deceived into thinking you need a vaginal deodorant, that's number eight. Using some kind of hair product? Now we're up to nine fragrances synthesized in industrial labs, and we still haven't put on the perfume or cologne that we intend for the world to inhale whenever we walk into a room. That's number ten.

Now let's get dressed—meaning we'll add in the aroma of our laundry detergent and maybe our dryer sheet or fabric softener, too. That's eleven and twelve. Almost forgot—currently, something called an "in-wash scent booster" is popular, just in case our clothing needs to smell even better than we do.

That's more than a dozen different chemical smells. Which one is us? None of the above. What *do* we smell like? Who knows? Maybe we smell great without all that stuff, but as long as we keep using it, we'll never know.

I get it, we'd all like our hair to smell like a tropical rain forest, even though not many of us know what a tropical rain forest actually smells like. And who doesn't want armpits that remind them of a field of wild lavender in the south of France? But come on! We're exposing ourselves to who-knows-what dangers just so we can smell like something we're not. Is that worth risking our health?

Now we're at home, another amazing convenience. It protects us from the harsh elements. It contains all the things we want and need to live (including all our other conveniences). It's the place we gather, where we can hang out for hours on end, sleep, make love, or do anything else we want—it's our castle. Once upon a time it was just a cave or a hut, but we've come a long way since then, and everything about our homes has only gotten better.

No wonder we love being there! But of course—as I've already said—every convenience comes with a price tag, whether we see it or not.

How is your house bad for your health? For one thing, our bodies and minds benefit from being outdoors in the open air, soaking up sunlight—in nature, because *we're* nature. And when we're outdoors, it's likely that we're moving around, and being in motion is another thing we need on a daily basis. Instead, we live more than 90 percent of our lives inside.

Indoors, we spend too much time sitting in chairs, hunched over computers, earning a living, meaning we're also courting back pain, neck pain, postural strain. When we had to hunt, gather, or grow our daily sustenance, we spent most of our waking hours outside. Inside was where we went once the sun set, and since there was no electricity for lamps, TVs, or video games and we were exhausted anyway, we went to sleep. Our waking and sleeping were dictated by the planet's rotation around the sun, our circadian sleep rhythms, and our biological clocks.

Besides pushing against our more natural rhythms by spending so much of our time indoors, there is the added risk of our homes being filled with furnishings and carpeting that have been treated with various noxious chemicals. Our furniture's upholstery and the lumber beneath it have probably been dosed with fire retardants and other chemicals. That sounded like a good idea when smoking was common and people had the unhealthy habit of dozing off on the sofa with a lit cigarette. We could have just resolved to be more careful, but instead we clamored for upholstery and even pajamas that had been treated with flame-retardant chemicals—without first checking to find out whether those chemicals caused health problems of their own.

Your carpeting? It was possibly treated with formaldehyde, a carcinogen. The paint on your walls? That also contains chemicals that put your health at risk. The sheetrock? All the glues used in your floor, whether it's tile or wood or something else? The same. Even those candles you love for how they fill your rooms with the aroma of the fake outdoors? That's not all they fill your rooms with.

The thing that happens is called *off-gassing*. The technical term is *volatile organic compounds*, or VOCs. It refers to the fumes that are constantly being given off by the objects we surround ourselves with. You can't see them, but if you can smell them, they're there. On any given day in our cozy homes, we might be gassed with formaldehyde, toluene, benzene, ammonia, and other nasty chemicals. You're inhaling all that stuff. It's entering through your nose, passing through your sinuses, and being sucked down into your lungs. That nice smell is created by those weird chemicals. They're inside you now.

We move from one controlled, artificial environment—our air-conditioned homes—into another—our air-conditioned cars and offices.

When's the last time you got good and sweaty? We've gotten to where we're horrified by the thought—is that a perspiration mark on my shirt? Am I giving off a slightly human smell? That's why antiperspirants were invented: to take the worry out of being close, as the commercials used to say.

To be honest, I'm not worried about being close. If I'm a healthy human being wearing clean clothing, there's nothing offensive about me. You, either. Nobody worried about being close until some clever adman thought it up, and he did so not out of concern for your social standing but so his boss could sell you a product containing aluminum salts, which stop the sweat from exiting your pores. Did he worry about the fact that those aluminum salts build up inside your body? And that aluminum has been linked to cancer and Alzheimer's disease? Probably not.

You want something to worry about? Try that.

Once, kids in particular had a strong connection to their wild nature. They spent as much time as possible outdoors, under the sun, running and playing together, having fun. But look at how the Fatal Convenience of home has changed their lives over the past few decades. Today you're more likely to find children and adolescents indoors, playing video games, burrowing into their apps, surfing the web, scrolling on their phones— exposing themselves to all kinds of radiation instead of the sun's rays.

Rather than sheltering in the comforts of our office or home all day long, we should take a break and go bask in sunlight to restore our vitamin D. It's crucial to our health, and many of us are deficient in it. Sure, we could take a vitamin supplement instead—and just pray that it's responsibly sourced and manufactured.

But keep in mind that nutritional supplements are more or less unregulated, which is why that industry has been described as the Wild West. We can't know for sure what's in those pills, capsules, or powders, no matter what the label says. In some cases, studies have shown, the supplement contains absolutely none—not a single molecule—of whatever its label says it is. On the other hand, we know what's in sunlight and all the benefits it has for us and every other living thing.

Maybe you've been told that sunlight is hazardous to your skin and too much exposure could lead to cancer. That's true in some cases. But the usual remedy—slathering on sunscreen—may not be any safer. Sunscreen can contain toxic or even carcinogenic ingredients that will do more damage than the sun will. Here's an idea: get some sunlight every day, but limit yourself to half an hour, either before or after the sun is at its highest point in the sky. There—problem solved without the "benefit" of a Fatal Convenience.

Now let's look at our food. Today, you can sit on your sofa, pick up your phone, order pretty much anything imaginable, and have it delivered to your door. You can expend zero calories in the effort to acquire meals fit for a king—several kings, in fact. That in itself is a disruption of the balance that exists everywhere in nature: every creature must expend energy in order to consume energy. Every creature except one.

Once upon a time we had to go out and forage or kill our food. Today, you can sit on your sofa and summon it with your phone. What kind of food? I'll take a guess that it's not nearly as wholesome or nutritious as what you might have cooked for yourself. But it sure is convenient.

Of course, we wouldn't want to have to grow or raise or hunt everything we eat. Nobody wants to go back to preagricultural days or to a time when if we liked bread, cheese, or wine, we had to make our own. But—as often happens with us humans—we went from doing everything for ourselves to doing nothing. All the food-related conveniences, starting with the development of farming thousands of years ago, have made our lives easier and allowed us to survive without the threat of starvation. Can't complain about that. But then we took our love of convenience too far.

We have a way of doing that. It comes up over and over in this book.

Drive down any highway in America, and you'll come upon food that is sold on the promise of how quickly the restaurant can get it into your belly—fast food. Does it taste good? To a lot of people, yeah, obviously. Keep in mind, corporations hire armies of food scientists to develop items that will send our taste buds into a frenzy of excitement and flood our brains with dopamine. That's their job.

But is the food good for us? Can we even call it food? Let's put it this way—caring about that is *not* the food engineers' job. The only people whose job it is to care about the quality of the food we eat are you and me.

I don't plan to be yet another person nagging you to stop eating things you love. But I do want you to pay attention to the Fatal Convenience that's at the heart of all junk food and see what it's doing to you.

A study published in the *Journal of the American Medical Association* found that around two-thirds of the calories consumed by American kids today are in the form of ultraprocessed foods, meaning the cheap and easy things that children—who don't know any better—love to eat; foods devoid of anything beneficial and full of nutritional nightmares.

Of course, kids don't have any money to go shopping, so they're not to blame. We adults are—we and the systems we support that allow these atrocities. Childhood obesity is at an all-time high and still rising, and by the time the youths of today are adults, they'll be dealing with that plus type 2 diabetes, which will bring with it a whole raft of debilitating diseases. That's not such a great inheritance to leave to our kids.

As if that weren't bad enough, Food and Drug Administration (FDA) testing recently found that the most popular brands of baby food include dangerously high levels of inorganic arsenic in the rice, exceeding the legal limits. And that's what we're feeding our kids? Imagine the junk that's in what the rest of us eat.

But hey, that ultraprocessed food sure is ultraconvenient! You don't have to cook it or do anything else with it to make it taste good, and there's no cleaning up afterward. Sure, the food corporations work tirelessly to make those foods hyperpalatable—better tasting than anything found in nature, so good they're addictive. But that's only part of their appeal. If they weren't so effortless to serve up, they wouldn't be nearly as popular. Why work if you don't have to?

HERE'S A SCARY THOUGHT: We don't have to use a single Fatal Convenience for their harmful contents to make their way into our bodies. Their junk is in the air we breathe and the food and water we consume. Thousands and thousands of industrial chemicals. Pesticides. Plastic residue. Metals. Hormone disruptors. The microparticles that every product sheds.

I recently read that the average human being consumes 200,000 tiny pieces of plastic every year! I bet you didn't know that, and how could you? Those little bits of petroleum-based nonbiodegradable garbage are invisible to the naked eye and tasteless, too. But they're inside you now, doing who knows what damage. Research has shown that microplastic consumption is partly responsible for the frightening plunge in global sperm counts. Even the living creatures who will never use a single Fatal Convenience are suffering. In the middle of the Pacific Ocean, dead albatrosses have been found with entire plastic bottles inside their bodies.

Remember that plastic water bottle you threw away two years ago? No? Well, that bottle remembers you—because by now it has entered into your environment in one form or another. It's begun to break down and leave tiny traces of plastic somewhere, perhaps in the ocean, meaning that it's inside the fish and will soon be inside you, too. That single-use bottle was such a great convenience. It meant you didn't have to bother carrying a reusable flask around all day. No refilling required. No lugging.

When you were done with that bottle, you threw it away and it was gone for good. But in fact there's no such thing as throwing anything away. There's no such thing as *away*. All our trash, especially the non-biodegradable junk, all our exhaust and effluents, all our residues and runoffs, maybe we can no longer see them. But they're there. They're *here*. This may be the worst offender of all the Fatal Conveniences, because it's the accumulation of every convenience we've ever enjoyed. We're literally drowning in all our poor decisions.

But hang on—how bad can any of those conveniences be when we have so many federal, state, and local agencies in place to protect us? The FDA, the CDC, the NIH, the EPA, the FTC, the USDA . . . the list of acronyms is endless. All are staffed with scientists, experts, and bureaucrats whose job it is to make sure we're not exposed to anything dangerous in our food or other consumer products.

However, as I just said, of the more than eighty thousand chemicals in commercial use today, most were untested before they reached us, and more than a thousand can cause cancer. But that doesn't mean they're automatically prohibited for human use. Every so often, scientific evidence of the danger of one of these substances will become impossible for governmental agencies to ignore. At that point, if we're lucky, it will be banned from the products that we use. Of course, by then we've been exposed to it for years—decades, even.

Here's a perfect example of this madness: in 2022, the federal government banned the use of a common crop pesticide called chlorpyrifos because research showed that it is linked to reduced IQ, lower birth weight, and other developmental problems in children. In some cases, the exposure started when the victims were fetuses, even before they were born.

But that's not the scariest part. This chemical has been in widespread use since 1965, meaning that several generations of kids were exposed to it before the government decided to take action. And right up until it was banned, there were lobbyists who fought against taking it off the market! Keep that in mind when you wonder whether we're really being legally fed poisons—even long after it's known that they're poisonous.

That's the only way government "protects" us. A manufacturer is not required to prove that a product or a chemical is safe before it goes into use. Only when the evidence of its danger is overwhelming and impossible to ignore will the government ban it. And even then, only maybe—and decades too late to do us much good. The mere fact that the government bans products that are already on the market tells us something frightful: nobody fully tests these substances *before* they reach us. It takes a lot of time, effort, and study before something that is proven to be bad for us actually goes away. Meanwhile, we're eating it, applying it to our skin, or feeding it to our children—totally unaware of the harm it's doing.

Relying on governmental agencies and bureaucrats to protect us is itself a seductive, dangerous Fatal Convenience. It's easy to believe that somebody else is looking out for us. It's the most passive approach to health that I can think of—like waiting for a cavalry that always arrives too late to save the day. This chemical is possibly cancer causing? Gee, thanks for letting us know—ten years after we started using products that contain it.

We go through life behaving as though we're being protected from harm, for the simple reason that to live otherwise—to accept the fact that we have to protect ourselves—is too scary to think about. The idea that we need to stop and worry about every single thing we put into or onto our bodies and then investigate all the various substances that go into them before we can use them . . . we'd all have to become full-time scientific investigators. We wouldn't have time to do anything else.

So we cross our fingers and hope that if it is on store shelves, it must be safe, and if anything was really and truly poisonous, we'd know about it. We'd see people falling ill all around us. Since that hasn't happened, we believe that everything sold at the supermarket really is "food" and even the stuff we call junk food isn't doing us irreparable harm. Or we assume that everything sold in a drugstore is beneficial to our health and does exactly what it says on the label and nothing more—nothing bad.

Dream on.

It's crazy that we have to remind ourselves that many of those products exist because businesses have figured out our deepest insecurities, vanities, and fears and come up with ways to exploit them for profit. Their profits are more important than our health.

We need to be sure that something is safe *before* we let it into our lives. We have to take a close look at our conveniences, question their purpose, and wonder what they might be doing to us.

Really—interrogate everything!

That sounds a little comical, I realize. But I'm honestly suggesting that tomorrow morning you look at your tube of toothpaste and, before you brush, read the list of ingredients. Then ask it, "What are you *really*? What are you putting inside my mouth? How much are you helping me? Are you truly the best I can do?"

Then look down at your carpet and ask it, "What the heck is in *you*? Are you friend or foe?" When you get the answer, you might discover that the nice, soft rug that feels so good under your bare feet has been exhaling formaldehyde into your face all along. Holy cow!

Next, you can interrogate your sheets. Your microwave oven. Your laundry detergent. Your deodorant. Come right out and ask it, "Do I even *need* you? Do I *have* a bad odor? Because when I stop and think about it, *I don't stink!*"

In many cases, I predict, you'll examine something you've been using forever and realize that you don't need it at all. That's automatically an improvement! Plus, you'll save money.

It sounds like work, I know. We have become so accustomed to the conveniences in our lives that they've become like old friends—we can't even remember how we met or why we hit it off. It's as though they've been there forever.

When I went away to college, I immediately started using the same laundry detergent my mom had always used. Who better than your mother to tell you how to clean your clothes? And they came out smelling the way they always had, which comforted a homesick college kid. If I hadn't wised up along the way, I might still be using the same detergent my mother used back in the 1970s, even though it's probably filled with the toxic chemicals I try so hard to avoid. In fact, there's no guarantee that her brand of detergent is still made using the same formulation, even though the name is unchanged. Over the course of years, corporations find different (usually cheaper) ingredients to use. Do they announce the changes? Of course not. They want it to seem like the same wholesome product it's always been.

I can say the same about every kind of commercial big-brand product—foods, beverages, skin care products, clothing, soap, cologne, all of it. We're buying a name, and beyond that—who knows *what* we're buying?

Once we begin really examining the conveniences in our lives, we'll become more aware, involved participants in our own well-being. We'll get back some of the sovereignty over our existence that we have given away to companies and products that really, let's face it, don't care about our health as much as they care about their own profits.

But even if we take the time to interrogate our conveniences, we're not scientists—most of us, at least. How can we know what's safe and what's not? Here's a good general rule: we are all living creatures, created by nature, so everything in our lives should be, too—or as much as possible. You don't have to be a biologist to know that pure, organic coconut oil is closer to your biology—and more effective at moisturizing your skin—than a fancy skin lotion with a dozen ingredients, most of which you don't recognize or can easily pronounce.

A good first question to ask whenever we're considering any product: Is it found in nature, more or less in this form? If the answer is yes, it's probably safe. (Though even that isn't always the case.) If the answer is no, proceed with caution.

I know what you're probably thinking: "How much bodily damage am I *really* doing with that little bit of formaldehyde I inhale every day? Who has actually gotten cancer from the Teflon in their no-iron shirts or had their hormones seriously disrupted by their mascara? Can't we just not worry about *one thing*? I'm already anxious enough!"

Honestly? You're partly right; it's not possible to accurately measure the damage done by daily exposure to *all* the harmful substances we come into contact with. You can't easily tease out the impact on our bodies—there are too many variables. So it's possible to rationalize our worries away by thinking that each tiny assault on our health probably isn't such a big deal.

But we don't get them separately, in tiny bits. We get them all together, each one piled on top of the other. We absolutely do know for a fact that we're exposing ourselves to multiple hazardous substances every day, all day.

Here's the question, then: At what point does a single straw break the poor camel's back?

Lately, scientists have come up with a new way to think about these questions; they call it *cumulative body burden*, meaning the combined effects of all the substances we come into contact with during the course of daily living. It's a way to show how our health is affected not just by one substance but by all of them together—the way we actually take them in. More important, it shows that once we absorb harmful chemicals, they don't go anywhere in a hurry. They linger inside our bodies and mingle with our tissues.

We got a lesson in total body burden from an unexpected source. Scientists used to believe that developing fetuses were protected from toxins and pollution by the mother's placenta. But then, according to a 2005 report issued by the Environmental Working Group (EWG), an activist group dedicated to research and advocacy:

> Researchers at two major laboratories found an average of 200 industrial chemicals and pollutants in umbilical cord blood from 10 babies born in August and September of 2004 in U.S. hospitals. Tests revealed a total of 287 chemicals in the group. The umbilical cord blood of these 10 children, collected by Red Cross after the cord was cut, harbored pesticides, consumer product ingredients, and wastes from burning coal, gasoline, and garbage.
>
> This study represents the first reported cord blood tests for 261 of the targeted chemicals and the first reported detections in cord blood for 209 compounds. Among them are eight perfluorochemicals used as stain and oil repellents in fast food packaging, clothes and textiles—including the Teflon chemical PFOA, recently characterized as a likely human carcinogen by the EPA's Science Advisory Board—dozens of widely used brominated flame retardants and their toxic by-products; and numerous pesticides.
>
> Of the 287 chemicals we detected in umbilical cord blood, we know that 180 cause cancer in humans or animals, 217 are toxic to the brain and nervous system, and 208 cause birth defects or abnormal development in animal tests. The dangers of pre- or post-natal

exposure to this complex mixture of carcinogens, developmental toxins and neurotoxins have never been studied.

Pretty awful, right? Even before we're born, we're carrying a full load of harmful, even poisonous substances that exist in our mother's surroundings and in the products she consumes.

Then, in 2008, the EWG examined the total body burden carried around by teenage girls. That study found sixteen substances, some of which have been linked to cancer and hormone disruption, in blood and urine samples taken from girls ages fourteen to nineteen. They included DDT, the pesticide that was banned in 1972; lead, which was phased out of gasoline starting in 1975; and the Teflon chemical PFOA.

Another important piece of the puzzle was revealed by the C8 Health Project. This was thanks to an environmental disaster, when the DuPont chemical company turned some West Virginia farmland into a toxic waste disposal site for poisons from a factory making chemicals used in Teflon and other industrial junk. Those waste products were found to be responsible for illnesses and deaths of people who lived nearby. They killed cattle and wildlife, too.

A legal settlement required DuPont to set up a research project to study the total effects of the chemicals—which are called per- and polyfluoroalkyl substances, or PFASs, but are also known as C8—on people living in the mid–Ohio Valley. The scientists released "probable link reports" indicating whether they did or did not find evidence that the chemical exposures caused various illnesses.

Guess what they found? Probable links to six different disease categories: kidney cancer, testicular cancer, thyroid disease, ulcerative colitis, pregnancy-induced hypertension, and high cholesterol levels.

Dr. Shanna H. Swan is one of the world's leading environmental and reproductive epidemiologists. She's a professor of environmental medicine and public health at the Icahn School of Medicine at Mount Sinai in New York City. Dr. Swan studies how chemicals in our environment and the products we use disrupt our reproductive systems, including the dramatic global drop in sperm count. She is the author of a landmark book titled *Count Down: How Our Modern World Is Threatening Sperm Counts, Altering Male and Female Reproductive Development, and Imperiling the Future of the Human Race*, published in 2021.

I asked her about the effects of all the toxic substances accumulating in our bodies. "The question of cumulative body burden is complicated," she said. "The chemicals that are nonpersistent (like the phthalates and bisphenols—think BPA) do not accumulate. They have short half-lives (four to six hours), but the exposure is ongoing. It comes into our bodies from the foods and products we are exposed to every day. On the other hand, the persistent EDCs (endocrine-disrupting chemicals, such as dioxins, PCBs, and so on) have long half-lives and do accumulate in body fat. In between those are the semipersistent ones, such as flame retardants and the PFAS chemicals, which have half-lives of many days.

"Aside from accumulation," she went on, "there is the issue of mixtures. We are exposed to over a hundred chemicals at once on an ongoing basis. And their joint effects are often greater than predicted by their individual risk, as is the case with medications, which is why your physician wants to know everything you are taking before she prescribes a new drug.

"Finally, there is the cumulative effect across generations. Patricia A. Hunt [a professor in the School of Molecular Bioscience at Washington State University, best known for showing the effects of bisphenol A on the reproductive system] has shown that exposure to EDCs in consecutive generations magnifies the damage. It's not as if each generation started with a clean slate; the parents' and even grandparents' exposure affects their offspring in a cumulative way.

"Bottom line," Dr. Swan concluded, "the unborn fetus is exposed in all these ways, and these exposures permanently affect his/her in utero development and future health and function. Then, after birth, exposure continues and acts on top of the in utero exposure."

Staggering! Let me sum it all up: Some harmful chemicals last in our bodies for just a few hours. But we're exposed to them constantly, so they never really go away. Other bad stuff hangs around much longer, in our body fat, continuously causing damage as long as it's there. The big risk is that these toxins interact and become even more dangerous in combination—and so powerful that we can pass the harm along in our genes to future generations.

That's scary shit, I know.

My goal in writing this book isn't to frighten you away from the conveniences that make things easier, more practical, more pleasant. As I said before, I love conveniences as much as you do. I enjoy all the same ones as everybody else, trust me. The only difference is that I do my best to choose conveniences that won't do me harm. They aren't exposing me to chemicals that have proven to be carcinogenic, hormone disrupting, or bad for the environment—or to substances so new that we don't really know what their effect will be on our health down the line. The conveniences I use aren't constantly blasting me with electromagnetic radiation, cancer-causing pesticides, or endocrine system–altering lab concoctions.

Yet my skin, hair, and clothes are as well tended as anybody else's. I have a comfortable house full of the latest electronic equipment and gadgets, more than most people I know.

But I refuse to buy products that will make me sick or—I'm serious!—possibly kill me. I've written this book so you can say the same. My goal here is not just to call out Fatal Conveniences; it's to find solutions—better ways. Better Conveniences. Knowledge is power, and it's time we take it back.

2

THIS IS THE CHAPTER
ABOUT MY DAD

THE SUBJECT OF *FATAL CONVENIENCES* **MEANS** a lot to me, even beyond the obvious reason of wanting everybody to be safe and healthy. It's a story.

Back in the 1990s, when I was in college, my father started experiencing something weird. He was a university professor, an intellectual guy with a lot of empathy. Most of his life revolved around his intelligence and his ability to learn, reason, and teach. Suddenly he began having foggy mental episodes, when he couldn't think straight or focus. He felt as though he was losing it, and he didn't know why.

He went to physicians and even to a psychiatrist, but no one could explain what was happening. Finally, he was told he might have a "chemical sensitivity disorder," which they barely understood and didn't know how to treat. The experts believed that for some mysterious reason his neurological system had become incapable of handling the everyday substances in his surroundings—the same ones the rest of us dealt with without even noticing.

That caused a pretty dramatic change in his life. It was a kind of torture, really. It forced him to isolate himself from the rest of the world. He had to avoid situations where he might be near people who used any kind of personal care product that contained a fragrance—meaning soap, shampoo, deodorant, lotion, perfume. Oh, laundry detergent, too. It also meant that he had to stop using those things, so in the pre-Google era, he had to hunt for products that didn't contain the widely used chemicals that were making his life such misery. Try to imagine what it would be like to live that way. Virtually impossible. But for him the alternative was even worse—it was as though his brain could no longer function.

We didn't know what to make of it, naturally. All of a sudden, our dad couldn't be near us or anyone else? We all thought he was going crazy! He must have been in the grip of a mental disorder that he was blaming on invisible chemicals in the air. Who ever heard of such a thing? I was just a kid from Minnesota, and now my dad, who was a really smart guy, was telling us that the products we all used every day—the same things used by everybody else in the world—were harming him and, as far as we could tell, him alone.

Because he was a professor, a man of science, he did tons of research and gave us photocopies of articles and scientific papers, stapling them and highlighting the important parts. He made us VHS copies of videos, too, since that was all pre-YouTube. And he was telling us, as a family, "Hey, these things are toxic. They trip me out. Don't wear this stuff around me." He would give us each a care package—he'd say, "Here's the soap to use, here's the shampoo, here's the deodorant, here's the toothpaste, here's the whatever. And you can't wear clothes that you just washed, because you didn't use the right laundry detergent. And you can't use cologne or aftershave or anything like that." All those restrictions were like layers separating him from his family and the rest of the world. We knew he was suffering, and of course we wanted to hang out with him. But it wasn't easy.

At the same time, he was trying to maintain his career, switching from professor to counselor, though that still meant that he would have contact with other people. And the same issues came up. He had to send letters to everyone he knew, saying "Hey, listen, I have this thing, it's called chemical sensitivity. These deodorants, these shampoos, these fragrances, they all fog me out, so could you please not wear them when you're seeing me, and here are some alternatives."

You can imagine how that went over. Nobody knew what he was talking about. It just drove him deeper into himself and away from everybody else. It was a downward spiral into isolation and depression.

I have another memory of my dad, from when I was even younger—when I was a kid and he was telling me about his time in the US Navy. He had been part of a select group called "Keepers of the Dragon," specialists who maintained and kept control of our nuclear bombs. He was aboard one of the aircraft carriers used to blockade Cuba during the 1962 missile crisis, when we nearly went to nuclear war with the Soviet Union. He had been exposed to radioactivity, which settles in the thyroid gland and can cause cancer. The only treatment was to swallow radioactive isotopes, which travel to the gland and actually destroy it.

So that was what the doctors prescribed, and he was on thyroid medication for the rest of his life. Could that have been the cause of his chemical sensitivity? When you mess with the endocrine system, you mess with everything else in the body. Was that to blame? I'll never know for sure. But I suspect that it had to have affected him.

Eventually his disability forced him to retire from the university, which only deepened his isolation and made him more depressed. Even he began to wonder, "What's *really* wrong with me? What is going on inside my head?" Doctors prescribed drugs they thought would bring back his ability to focus and lift some of the mental fog. None of it helped. Before long, my dad, who had suffered years before from alcohol addiction, was taking multiple prescription medications, Ritalin and others, more than any of his doctors knew. Then, after thirty years of being sober, he began drinking again. His chemical sensitivity issues had started him down a path where everything quickly went wrong.

Eventually, he died of alcoholism. But that wasn't what really killed him.

SOMETHING UNEXPECTED CAME OUT OF that sad time. Because of my dad, I had stopped using products with chemicals that triggered him. It was the only way we could spend time together. As a result, *I* became sensitive to the same things that plagued him. Not in the extreme way he was affected—I could still think and focus just fine. But it was as though I had gone through chemical detox. Suddenly, I couldn't stand being around people who used normal soaps and shampoos and lotions and so on. I was in my twenties at that point, in college, so you can imagine what it was like to go through life trying to avoid exposure to the common products everybody else used.

But when I was near someone wearing perfume or aftershave, it was as though I had been punched in the face. I felt assaulted. As long as I continued using the products my dad had introduced me to, I felt great. Healthy. Clear-headed. To this day, if someone comes around me wearing anything with a strong fragrance, it feels intrusive—perfume, cologne, new-car smell, scented candles, most soaps, the same.

That experience opened my eyes. If you saw any of the *Matrix* movies, you know the meaning of the red pill. The Keanu Reeves character is offered a choice: take the blue pill or the red pill. The blue pill will allow him to go on living in comfortable blindness to the reality of the world around him. If instead he takes the red pill, he will suddenly see the truth of his existence—that everything he thought was real was a lie, created to keep people from knowing that they're living inside a simulated world manufactured by evil machines.

He takes the red pill. Pow!

That's how it felt to me—like giving up all those products had opened my eyes to a shocking truth: that the most common conveniences, the ones we all used and enjoyed, were doing us harm. They contained chemical substances and other things that had been created in labs, and because those substances were invisible, we had no idea that we were being constantly bathed in them, twenty-four hours a day, for our entire lives.

That's *our* Matrix: the invisible fog of synthetic chemicals, electromagnetic radiation, petroleum by-products, microplastics, pesticides, hormone disruptors, and all the other harmful junk that surrounds us. Most of us inhabit it without ever suspecting a thing. We get sick and even die, and we never know why.

That's the world of Fatal Conveniences. We think we're seeing reality. We believe that our homes, our food, our clothes, and all the products we buy and use to make our lives easier exist for our benefit, with no downside.

Then, one day, we're offered the red pill.

Boom! Now we look around and see what was kept hidden from us all these years.

Today, the rest of the world is just beginning to catch up with my father. We're starting to realize how heavily we're being dosed with all kinds of gnarly chemicals. We're finally ready to face the truth.

Fortunately, there is a whole new world of consumer products being made with our well-being and the health of our planet in mind. Every day I hear about new choices—in everything from skin care to clothing to household products to consumer electronics. We now have alternatives to the poisonous garbage out there. In these pages, once I expose all the conveniences that are doing us harm, I'm going to talk about the products that perform the same functions.

But without killing us.

3

OUR CHEMICAL ROMANCE

YOU'RE GOING TO NOTICE, AS YOU read this book, that I spend a lot of time talking about chemicals. Not the most exciting subject to many, I suspect, but it's important to understand, at least a little, if we're going to deal with all the dangers constantly swimming around us. I'll try not to turn this into homework.

First, let me point out something obvious: everything contains chemicals. Water and air are made of chemicals. Trees, grass, and flowers are made of chemicals. Puppies, kittens, and bunnies are made of chemicals. Your mom is made of chemicals!

And just because a chemical is found in nature doesn't mean it's safe or healthy. Rice, for example, contains arsenic. Every year people die from poisonous mushrooms. Salt, if you eat too much, will kill you. Some minerals are radioactive.

But it's the nonnatural chemicals that should worry us, the new ones that are constantly being created in industrial labs for commercial uses. There are more than eighty thousand in existence and more being created every year, only a small number of which (medicines and pesticides, mostly) are ever tested for safety. Neither does anyone test them to see how they interact with one another.

Let that sink in: these substances are out in our world, we're all being exposed to them every minute of every day, yet for a long time nobody in charge thought it was a good idea to evaluate them first to see if they would make us sick or kill us.

How could that be?

In truth, there were plenty of scientists who believed that chemicals should be tested. But big business and lax regulators made sure that didn't happen. This situation began to change a little in 1976, when a federal law, the Toxic Substances Control Act, was passed. But it took four more decades before that law was given some teeth, with the 2016 passage of a reform bill, the Frank R. Lautenberg Chemical Safety for the 21st Century Act. This gave the EPA the power to require testing of new and existing chemicals to see if they are harmful to our health. There are even some extra protections in there for children and pregnant women. But regulators are going to be playing catch-up for a long time, trying to test all existing chemicals along with the hundreds of new ones added annually.

The fact that these chemicals are, for the most part, invisible and undetectable means that we are unaware of what we're taking in with our food and water, the air we breathe, our personal care products, our clothing, and just about everything else we consume. Add in all the chemicals used in industrial processes that take place where we can't see them but still enter our environment, and the picture becomes even scarier. We're virtually helpless to defend ourselves.

Of course, that's government's main job—to keep us safe from forces beyond our control. But please don't go through life thinking that we can trust regulators to protect us from harm. For instance, at least three federal government agencies regulate the use of benzene, a carcinogen that's been linked to leukemia, bone marrow cancer, and other serious blood disorders. It's found in cigarette smoke and gasoline, which tells you how safe it must be.

Still, as I was writing this, a manufacturer announced the recall of eighteen varieties of a popular spray deodorant, all of which had concerning levels of the chemical. And a few months before that, another consumer products giant had to recall two of its sunscreens due to their benzene content.

What does this tell us? That even when the government tries to protect us, its efforts sometimes fail—and we don't find out until after the damage is done.

Testing individual chemicals isn't enough, because that doesn't evaluate how they behave in combination. It's possible that when two or more chemicals interact, they affect us in ways that neither one does on its own. Is it even possible to measure the infinite number of likely chemical combinations inside each one of us?

Nope!

In a 2015 study published in the journal *Carcinogenesis*, eighty-five commonly used industrial chemicals found in everyday products were tested to see if they could trigger cancerous tumors. Fifty of the chemicals were found to affect cancer-causing processes in the human body, even at the low levels found in our environment.

"We live in a chemical soup," said the toxicologist Linda Birnbaum, the then director of the National Institute of Environmental Health Sciences.

It seems to me that we have our priorities upside down. Corporations create products using untested chemicals, many of which are known to be harmful to human health. The companies grab the cash today, and when the scientific truth catches up with them, they ask for forgiveness, settle lawsuits, pay fines, and conduct product recalls. To them, this is just the cost of doing business, which is passed along to consumers. Human safety is not their top priority. Our health is not their responsibility. That's the truth.

Let's look at just one group of man-made substances that's everywhere in our lives. Their scientific name is PFAS, or in some cases PFOS, though both are also known as "forever chemicals." That nickname is a pretty good hint about why we should fear them.

I won't bore you with any of the technical jargon used to describe these industrial concoctions, but I will point out that they've been deemed by scientists as "persistent organic pollutants," and it's the *persistent* part that should worry us. It means that they endure, without breaking down, for a very long time, in the environment—and also inside us.

PFAS chemicals make surfaces slick and frictionless. That's pretty much all they do. You might not imagine that making things slippery would be such a huge industry, with so many applications. But it definitely is. These chemicals are why some fabrics don't wrinkle, why your mascara is waterproof, why fast food doesn't stick to the wrapper, and why dental floss slips so easily between your teeth, to name just a few of the hundreds of commercial uses.

The most famous of these chemicals, Teflon, the nonstick surface on cookware, was developed by a DuPont scientist in the 1940s. A decade later, the stain repellent Scotchgard was discovered in a 3M lab—by accident. (An experimental compound spilled on a lab assistant's sneaker, and that spot refused to get dirty.) By 2000, Scotchgard was a $300-million-a-year product, but it was around that time that 3M realized that the active chemicals were, in the words of a researcher in *Environmental Science and Technology*, "persistent, bioaccumulative, ubiquitous in the environment and linked with adverse effects in laboratory experiments," meaning that they were long lasting, widespread, and dangerous—an ugly combination.

At that point, the company developed other formulations so that Scotchgard could continue to do its job. But stain repellents are still the biggest use of these chemicals, with an estimated global market of over $2 billion a year. Teflon is no longer used in nonstick coating. But cousins of Teflon still show up hidden inside many products we all wear and use.

I'd love to offer you a complete list of all these forever chemicals so you can avoid them. But I can't—according to the federal Environmental Protection Agency, there are by now thousands of them in circulation. And nowhere on any label will you ever find the acronym PFAS, so don't bother looking. The different ways in which we are exposed to these chemicals is so long, it will make you dizzy. Here's just a partial list of where they're found:

Stain-resistant fabrics
Lipstick, eyeliner, mascara, foundation, concealer, lip balm,
  and blush
Nail polish
Firefighting foam
Baby bibs
Bedding
Carpets
No-iron clothing
Waterproof outerwear
Furniture and car upholstery
Fast-food wrappers
Plastic food packaging
Microwave popcorn
Leather
Paper
Rubber

Thanks to all those products (and more!), these chemicals are widely dispersed throughout our environment, which is how our tap water has become contaminated with them. And when our drinking water contains something, we do, too. The US Centers for Disease Control and Prevention (CDC) says it has found PFASs in the blood of nearly every individual it has tested for them, indicating "widespread exposure to these PFAS in the U.S. population."

So unless you've been living in a cave on a mountaintop near a bubbling spring far from civilization for the past fifty years, you definitely have these chemicals in your body. If you're pregnant, your developing baby has some, too, despite the fact that he or she has yet to enjoy any conveniences of any kind.

Their potential for harm isn't even slightly in question. An advisory board to the EPA called them a "likely" carcinogen in humans. According to the Environmental Working Group, "The PFAS pollution crisis is a public health emergency." PFASs have been linked to:

+ Kidney cancer
+ Testicular cancer
+ Liver disease
+ Thyroid disease
+ High cholesterol levels
+ Ulcerative colitis
+ Difficulties during pregnancy
+ Suppressed immune system in children
+ Low birth weight

In the summer of 2021, the US House of Representatives passed the PFAS Action Act, which would allow the EPA to limit the chemicals' presence in drinking water, require testing of every PFAS for toxicity, and force all consumer products labels to list these chemicals when they are among the ingredients. If it had been enacted into law, it would have made a difference, we're told. But it died in Congress. The best we can expect, it seems, is that the current White House will do everything in its power to eliminate PFASs from our lives. That's definitely not all we could hope for. It's absolutely less than we need and deserve. But it's better than nothing, I guess.

But while we're waiting (and *waiting*) for action on that legislation, no limits have been set on the concentration of PFASs in our drinking water, as they have for other pollutants such as benzene, uranium, and arsenic. Tired of depending on the feds, seven states—California, Connecticut, Maine, Minnesota, New York, Vermont, and Washington—have banned them. Eight other states—Colorado, Hawaii, Iowa, Maryland, Massachusetts, Michigan, Pennsylvania, and Rhode Island—have proposed similar legislation.

Can we do anything else about them? We can all invest in water filters, true, and make every effort to protect ourselves. But that's not a real solution to a societywide disaster.

Manufacturers have agreed to phase out some PFASs used in food packaging by 2024. Some of the biggest fast-food outfits, including McDonald's, Wendy's, Chipotle, and Panera Bread, have promised to stop using wrappers lined with PFASs. In 2021, legislation called the Keep Food Containers Safe from PFAS Act was introduced in both houses of Congress.

Unfortunately, PFASs will still come into the country in goods imported from abroad. Again, the fact that these are "forever" chemicals means that the ones in existence now aren't going away soon. Maybe future generations will benefit from these steps. But if you're alive today, PFASs are in your system.

There's a lesson here: the sweeter the convenience, the greater the potential harm it's capable of causing. How much time and effort have we saved thanks to no-iron sheets, nonstick frying pans, stain-resistant fabric? Was it worth the potential of developing cancer, hormone disruption, and all the other ills associated with PFASs? Not to me. But to the companies that created all these so-called miracles? The profits tell the tale.

Another danger of forever chemicals is that they are known hormone disruptors, meaning that they interfere with our endocrine system and even our ability to make babies. This is serious stuff; our hormones control not just our reproductive functions but also a long list of other systems that keep us alive and well. These chemicals are responsible for neutering boys by damaging their ability to produce sperm. They also can push girls into early puberty.

According to the National Institute of Environmental Health Sciences (NIEHS), a federal agency, endocrine disruptors are found in a long list of chemicals used to make products we buy and use in our homes, our clothing, even in the foods we eat. Here are just a few of the most common examples on the NIEHS list.

+ **Bisphenol A (BPA):** Used to make polycarbonate plastics and epoxy resins, which are found in many plastic products including food storage containers
+ **Dioxins:** Produced as a by-product of herbicide production and paper bleaching; are also released into the environment during waste burning and wildfires
+ **Perchlorate:** A by-product of the aerospace, weapons, and pharmaceutical industries found in drinking water and fireworks
+ **Phthalates:** Used to make plastics more flexible; found in some food packaging, cosmetics, water bottles, children's toys, and medical devices
+ **Polybrominated diphenyl ethers (PBDEs):** Used to make flame retardants for household products such as furniture foam and carpets
+ **Polychlorinated biphenyls (PCBs):** Used to make electrical equipment such as transformers and in hydraulic fluids, heat transfer fluids, lubricants, and plasticizers
+ **Triclosan:** May be found in some antimicrobial and personal care products, such as liquid bodywash

According to the NIEHS, "Even low doses of endocrine-disrupting chemicals may be unsafe. The body's normal endocrine functioning involves very small changes in hormone levels, yet we know even these small changes can cause significant developmental and biological effects. This observation leads scientists to think that endocrine-disrupting chemical exposures, even at low amounts, can alter the body's sensitive systems and lead to health problems."

But the agency acknowledges the impossibility of knowing for sure the ways we're being affected by these chemicals: "Because people are typically exposed to multiple endocrine disruptors at the same time, assessing public health effects is difficult."

So even when we're aware of the potential risks, nobody—not even the experts—can figure out precisely how we're being harmed or how seriously. Given all that, what, if anything, can *we* do?

As I'll say again and again in these pages, we need to interrogate our conveniences before we start using them, not years or decades later. We need to make sure we know exactly what they contain and how their contents might harm us. We can't rely on officials to do it. The government's power to protect citizens is limited, especially when it comes to regulating corporations and commercial products. Certainly, we can't expect the companies to warn us off their merchandise, even when they know or suspect the damage it will do. I wish this weren't true, but it's up to us to protect ourselves.

Many of the man-made chemicals contained in products that we buy every day are poisoning our air, water, soil, and bodies. This is not about consumerism or politics—it's pure common sense: the businesses we support shouldn't be harming us. But as we'll see, virtually every personal care product contains untested synthetic chemicals. The same is true of household soaps and detergents, as well as the clothes you and your family wear. And no one is responsible if some turn out to be toxic.

At some point down the line, somebody will say, "Gee, if only we had known it caused cancer or some other horrible disease!" We *did* know. At least some of us did. Official neglect is called "plausible deniability." It means that if a governmental agency or company didn't know for sure that a substance was harmful, how could they warn us about it? From my point of view, this is a crime.

How are we okay with this? And if we're not, why do we accept it?

Let's decide now that we are through living this way and demand change. Let's create a world that will allow us to live healthy lives, where businesses will take seriously their responsibility to do the right things for humans, animals, and the planet we all call home.

4

PERSONAL CARE PRODUCTS

OF ALL THE CATEGORIES OF FATAL CONVENIENCES, this is the one that really makes me shake my head. Maybe it's the term itself. These products claim to provide us with care for our most personal physical needs. Instead, they often do the exact opposite: they harm us and put us at risk, maybe not intentionally, by containing ingredients that either are untested or have been proven to be sketchy, irritating, toxic, even carcinogenic.

The fact that we buy these goods in pharmacies and stores devoted to beauty and well-being makes it even worse. It gives them a halo of health and wholesomeness, so we don't question whether they're necessary or good for us or even if they do what they say they will.

Try this: Pick out a random personal care product you own or one from a store shelf, then read the mind-boggling list of ingredients—those endless, scary chemical names in type so tiny it's almost illegible. Then ask yourself if they really sound like substances you want on your skin, in your mouth, close to your eyes, or near your children. But give those industrial chemicals a cool brand name, a soothing image on the container (green leaves, flowers, etcetera), a relaxing fragrance, and a crafty marketing plan, and we're all suckers.

Maybe we think that because these products are used mostly on our surfaces—our skin, hair, nails—that they can't do us much harm. They feel good and smell nice, and they make pretty promises, and that's about all we consider. We forget that our skin is a vital organ just like our lungs, our heart, or any other, and that it has an extremely important job: to protect our insides from all the bad stuff outside, the harmful microbes, pollution, and poisons and all the rest.

Or maybe we just think we're unacceptable unless we look, feel, and smell differently than we naturally do. A great many corporate fortunes have been built on exploiting human insecurity.

The average American woman uses twelve personal care products every day, exposing herself to as many as 126 unique chemicals. Some of them have been linked to cancers of the breast and female reproductive organs. Others are endocrine-system disruptors, causing early-onset puberty in girls—which is itself an increased risk factor for certain cancers later in life. Men are no better off; we use nearly as many products containing the same gnarly substances, putting ourselves at similar risk. Keep in mind something that I will bring up repeatedly: These chemicals join all the other toxic substances we're subjected to on a daily basis.

Finally, there's one more way personal care products damage our health. Pretty much everything I'll discuss in this chapter is sold in a plastic container. When we finish our shampoo, bodywash, or sunscreen, out goes the bottle. But where exactly does it go? Recycling is kind of a scam—it makes us feel good to think every bit of plastic is being repurposed instead of ending up in a landfill somewhere. But it doesn't always happen. Even recycling requires the use of fossil fuel as energy.

According to the EPA, nearly 15 million tons of plastic containers and packaging are generated annually in the United States, and a lot of that is made to contain the products that keep us clean, pretty, and smelling sweet. Your empty bottles are adding to the global devastation caused by plastic overload, so the more personal care products you use, the more nonbiodegradable waste you are creating. Imagine the mountains of single-use plastic junk our beauty habits contribute to the environment. The cleaner we get, the filthier our world becomes.

You can see why I think of this product category as "personal harm."

FATAL CONVENIENCE: MOISTURIZER

Nature makes sure our skin stays moist, and for good reason: our epidermis is the first line of defense against all the nasty stuff—the bad bacteria, viruses, and fungi, the toxins, the irritants, the UV rays—that surrounds us every second of our lives and causes infection, inflammation, and worse.

To keep it from becoming dry and cracked and easily breached, human skin has somewhere between 2,500 and 6,000 sebaceous glands per square inch. They produce sebum, which we think of as oil but is actually a waxy substance that lubricates the skin, retains its moisture, and helps maintain its integrity. After our teenage years, the body's production of sebum goes into decline, at which point we may seek a little outside help.

"Moisturizer" is kind of a misnomer: these products mainly keep our skin from losing the moisture that our bodies naturally provide. It's also a catchall phrase, since there are various types of lotions and creams, and they do their job in slightly different ways. But the basis is the same: a mixture of water, a substance (often glycerin) that retains moisture, and other chemicals that combine to keep our skin intact.

The big question in the personal care category is whether the substances we rub on our skin manage to penetrate to our insides. There are chemicals that absolutely *do* cross that barrier—think of transdermal patches used to transport medicines through the skin and into the bloodstream. If you think that moisturizers enter deeply into your skin, however, think again; we are not permeable when it comes to lotions and creams. After all, our skin's main job is to keep things *out* of our bodies.

There's not a lot of independent research into the pros or cons of moisturizers, which doesn't stop manufacturers from using all kinds of scientific-sounding brags to hype their products. You'll sometimes see terms such as "hypoallergenic," "all natural," or even "noncomedogenic," meaning the product won't cause pimples, but these claims are pretty much meaningless, since there are no standards to guarantee them. There might also be a list of vitamins the lotion contains, but we have no way of knowing how much is there or whether they do anything to improve our skin. But it sure sounds healthy.

The top two ingredients in most moisturizers, water and glycerin—which is technically a humectant, meaning it retains water—are harmless. But we can't say the same about the long list of other substances listed on the label.

For instance, there is research proving that parabens and phthalates, which mimic hormones, can enter the bloodstream. And these are frequently found in moisturizers. How can you tell? You have to look very, very closely for ingredients such as methylparaben, propylparaben, butylparaben, and ethylparaben, or for the phthalates most commonly used in personal care products, such as butyl benzyl phthalate, monobenzyl phthalate, dibutyl phthalate, mono-n-butyl phthalate, monoisobutyl phthalate, di-isodecyl phthalate, and diisononyl phthalate.

They sound scary, don't they? There is also polyacrylamide, which is added to moisturizers to bind the ingredients and is made from the chemical acrylamide, a possible carcinogen.

Vitamin A (also listed as retinyl palmitate, retinyl acetate, retinoic acid, or retinol) is often added to moisturizer and promoted as an anti-wrinkle agent. However, it might actually damage the skin: research shows that vitamin A can increase sun sensitivity and lead to burns. Sun exposure may also break down vitamin A to produce toxic free radicals that damage DNA.

Lactic acid is also sometimes added to moisturizer to exfoliate your skin and make it glow. However, that power means it can be irritating and make your skin feel like it's burning.

And as we shall see elsewhere in this chapter, anything containing "fragrance" or "parfum" is suspect simply because those terms tell us nothing about what's in them. Part of the pleasure of rubbing cream or lotion into our skin is the soothing scent that comes along for the ride. It's a hard habit to break, I know.

At some point in your life, you may have used perhaps the most effective skin barrier on the market: petroleum jelly, better known under the trade name Vaseline. Slather that on your hide, and nothing will get in *or* out. Babies with diaper rash are routinely coated with it, and it does the trick, allowing their delicate skin to heal undisturbed.

On the other hand—it's made from crude oil!

"Petroleum jelly" sounds like something you would use to lubricate heavy machinery. Covering our living, breathing skin with the same substance used to make gasoline and polyester pants doesn't sound like the smartest idea, does it? In truth, there's no research showing that petroleum jelly is harmful when applied to human skin. However, the process of refining petroleum into petrolatum can lead to its contamination with polycyclic aromatic hydrocarbons, or PAHs, which are classified as carcinogens.

My advice is to avoid any moisturizer, lotion, or cream with ingredients that you don't recognize. Think of how you choose your food, and take the same approach: feed your skin a healthy, all-natural diet.

How About the Environment?

Obviously, anything made with a crude oil–based product is polluting the planet, and we already burn enough fossil fuels. After petroleum jelly, lanolin is the best substance for holding in water, but it comes from sheep glands and must be extracted from their bodies—not a pain-free process—and for that reason alone should be shunned and stopped. And don't forget all those plastic bottles you go through.

Okay, So What Should We Do?

First, use less soap when washing yourself. You'll be doing your skin a favor, because you're washing your natural sebum away. There's a reason most soaps and bodywashes contain moisturizer: manufacturers know that their products are drying you out.

Second, see what happens if you skip the moisturizer for a day or two. You might not even notice a difference, in which case maybe you can live without it permanently.

Third, try drinking more water. Our skin becomes dry not only because we lack oils but because we don't replace the water that escapes from the cells.

If you still feel the need, try the simplest solutions first, such as natural oils. Organic coconut oil, which is safe and clean, will provide all you need to keep natural moisture in. It will do the job as well as anything you can buy in the drugstore—even better, because it's cleaner (it's also cheaper).

If that solution seems a little too basic, try a product made with fair-trade shea butter, a natural emollient that has been used for thousands of years in Africa. Increased demand has created an environmental threat to shea trees, which take fifteen to twenty years to bear the nuts that produce the butter. It's important to support fair trade practices, to ensure that both the environment and the people who cultivate the trees are treated ethically.

There's a terrific product called Waxelene Multi-Purpose Ointment (waxelene.com). Its cruelty-free ingredients include vitamin E oil, beeswax, organic rosemary oil, and organic soy oil. According to the brand, the beeswax is unbleached and raw, and it has anti-inflammatory, antibacterial, and antioxidant benefits.

Rosemary oil improves blood circulation and with its antibacterial properties works as a natural preservative. Natural unrefined vitamin E oil also has antioxidant and anti-inflammatory properties and helps protect skin. Another good brand is Goē Oil (jaobrand.com), made of twenty-eight plant, fruit, and flower oils. The good news is that there are many safe, healthy, sustainable skin moisturizers available, some of which are listed in chapter 10.

FATAL CONVENIENCES: BODYWASH AND SOAP

Soap literally keeps us alive.

According to the CDC, nine out of ten foodborne illness outbreaks in the United States are caused by contamination due to food workers not washing their hands. It's not a rare occurrence and is definitely nothing to take lightly: every year, 48 million Americans get sick from their food, 128,000 are hospitalized, and 3,000 die. Around one-third of all diarrhea-related sicknesses and one-fifth of respiratory infections could be prevented by handwashing alone.

None of that should be surprising—long before your parents told you to wash your hands before dinner, way back in 1400 BCE, Moses's big brother Aaron made sure to scrub his before performing temple services. It makes sense: our skin is constantly being assaulted by filth, pollution, toxic chemicals, harmful germs, and unknown substances. Obviously, washing regularly is a no-brainer.

But water alone isn't enough to cleanse us. Soap makes the difference by mixing with the oil-like sebum on our skin to release the grit and grime we collect all day and rinse it away. Unfortunately, we're not content to stop there; today we overuse soap and bodywash to the point where we are damaging both ourselves and our environment.

Ask yourself: Just how disgusting do you get in the course of an average day? Do you wind up covered in mud or oil or drenched in sweat? Probably not, but most of us lather up daily from head to toe as though we require an extreme level of intensive cleansing. Either that or we think we're in a soap commercial, where bubbles are always produced in crazy abundance.

Our brains have been washed.

One problem when we overdo the scrubbing is that we remove the lubricants our bodies produce to protect our skin and keep it supple and intact. Too much washing causes not just visible redness but also invisible cracks in the skin, which let in the very things we're trying to keep out. One study of health care workers found that irritating the skin by overwashing affects the natural microbial flora of the hands, increasing the presence of dangerous bacteria that can cause methicillin-resistant *Staphylococcus aureus* (MRSA) infections.

And while hand cleanliness is important, it's questionable whether we need to lather up the rest of our bodies in their entirety every single day. Some doctors suggest showering just a few times a week and using soap only on armpits, groin, and anywhere else that requires it (you're an adult, you can figure this out on your own).

Once, of course, the issue of personal cleanliness was less of an obsession than it is today. Before running hot and cold water and indoor plumbing, you can understand why our bathing habits might have been more relaxed. People made soap at home, using fats from either animals or vegetables mixed with an alkali, such as lye. It was an all-natural solution that—as we will see throughout this book—has since been replaced by commercial versions made with synthetic chemicals. And that's where the problems start.

Reading soap labels is a tricky endeavor because the ingredients have weird chemical names, even the ones that are plant based and benign. For example, Mrs. Meyer's Clean Day products contain these scary-sounding yet naturally derived surfactants: sodium lauryl glucose carboxylate and sucrose laurate (derived from sugar); sodium laurylglucosides hydroxypropylsulfonate, and disodium 2-sulfolaurate (from coconuts); and sodium cocoamphoacetate (from plants). So rather than trying to decipher complicated ingredient lists, it might be easier to look instead for the ingredients to avoid.

Check labels for:

PARABENS: Methylparaben, propylparaben, butylparaben, and ethylparaben are all parabens. Their antimicrobial properties help protect against microorganisms, essentially acting as a preservative to lengthen the shelf life of the soap. But they're not so good for us. Parabens are easily absorbed by our bodies and act as endocrine disruptors; a 2013 study found decreased fertility among women with parabens detected in their urine. Not only that, but research also found that butylparaben worked with other cell receptors to increase the growth of breast cancer cells.

PHTHALATES/FRAGRANCES: A 2022 study of 5,303 adults found that exposure to phthalates was associated with cardiovascular-related and all-cause mortality. Previous research has linked the chemicals to increases in premature births, gestational diabetes, obesity, breast and thyroid cancers, and infertility. Diethyl phthalate is used to make the scent in soaps last longer, but the FDA doesn't require listing individual fragrance ingredients. The only way to avoid it is to steer clear of *any* product that lists fragrance as an ingredient, unless it's marked phthalate free.

ANTIBACTERIALS: A 2001 study found that 76 percent of liquid soaps contained the antibacterial agent triclosan or triclocarban. The problem is part of the much bigger issue of our overuse of antibiotics: at a certain point, they lose their effectiveness, meaning that they won't work when we really need them. In 2013, the FDA banned the use of those two chemicals in soap. In response, manufacturers replaced them with different antibacterials, such as benzalkonium chloride, benzethonium chloride, and chloroxylenol, disturbing news since those chemicals have been an effective treatment option for drug-resistant staph infections. To top it off, there's no evidence that they do a better job than plain soap and water. But people respond to the "antibacterial" promise, and soap sellers are happy to oblige.

SODIUM LAURETH SULFATE: This is a common bodywash surfactant, not to be confused with sodium *lauryl* sulfate. The process of turning lauryl sulfate (which is known to be irritating to the skin) into laureth sulfate creates the cancer-causing chemical 1,4-dioxane as a by-product. However, the jury is not entirely out on sodium lauryl sulfate (SLS), a synthetic chemical usually derived from petroleum but that can also be derived from plants. According to research funded by the soap maker Seventh Generation, there is no scientific evidence that SLS is dangerous. And since it is biodegradable, it is unlikely to damage the environment. EWG seems to agree, giving the ingredient a low score of 1 to 2. I am not fully convinced.

How About the Environment?

A study examining the environmental effect of increased use of soap during the pandemic found that high concentrations of detergents in fresh water "can cause massive foam to be created on water's surface, leading to the reduced rate of oxygen penetration into water." That's bad news for aquatic animal and plant life. Soap runoff can also make its way from water to land, where it damages soil and plants.

Palm oil, a common ingredient in soap and other personal care products, is natural, but that's the problem. Its harvesting has been linked to tropical deforestation, peat land draining and burning, declines in biodiversity, greenhouse gas emissions, and air pollution. And "sustainable" palm oil may be a fantasy. According to a 2018 study, so-called sustainable palm oil extraction still resulted in wildlife habitat degradation and forest loss.

But as I said earlier, probably the worst effect of bodywash on the environment has zero to do with the soap itself—it's the plastic bottles that it comes in.

Okay, So What Should We Do?

Soap clearly serves an important purpose, but we must use it sensibly. Too much won't make you cleaner but could damage your skin and the environment. Get over the myth that you'll be a social pariah unless you scrub yourself until you shine.

Whenever practical, use bodywash instead of bar soap, for the emulsifiers that help lubricate your skin. Bodywash is basically the same thing as soap but usually contains emollients. Research shows that shea butter, soybean oil, and coconut oil help moisturize the skin and are gentler than harsh chemical products.

Look for products made with simple ingredients, as few as possible, and sold in environmentally friendly packaging.

FATAL CONVENIENCES: TOOTHPASTE, DENTAL FLOSS, AND MOUTHWASH

Many millennia ago, anthropologists tell us, people used twigs, feathers, animal bones, homemade rinses, and other oddities to clean their mouths. That's no surprise considering how important teeth and gums are to our overall health. For one thing, if you can't eat, you can't live.

Also, our mouths are the wide-open portals to our insides, so we had better defend them against harmful bacteria and other hazards. And as we've seen elsewhere in this chapter, the main reason to keep our hands clean is so they don't infect us through our mouths.

So your mouth is not just an orifice in the middle of your face—it's an environment, with its own ecology, and to ignore that fact is to ask for trouble.

On the other hand, to address it incorrectly can be almost as bad. Let me ask you something: Are your teeth pearly white? Is your breath minty fresh? Are your gums perfectly pink and just the right size? It's the insecurity stoked by the oral care industry that keeps the rest of us anxious about whether our mouths are a joy to behold or unsightly, foul-smelling sewers to be shunned.

It all falls under the universal human fear of smelling bad from one body part or another. Entire fortunes have been built on such terrors.

Let's take a look.

Toothpaste

Watch any toothpaste commercial. The stuff comes out of the tube creamy and white, maybe with colored stripes or even glitter, looking good enough to eat. It must take a lot of ingenuity (and industrial chemicals and processes) to make it look so delicious. But what does that have to do with oral health?

Most toothpastes contain chemicals that have zero to do with cleaning our teeth and gums. For instance: saccharin is there to make it sweet; sodium lauryl sulfate creates the bubbly foam we take as proof of cleaning power; blue covarine tricks the eye by changing the way light reflects off our choppers, making them appear less yellow and more white; activated charcoal scrubs really well but can damage enamel and doesn't make our teeth any whiter; triclosan is an antibacterial that actually increases our resistance to other antibiotics. The flavoring agents are there just to make toothpaste tasty, but would you really neglect your oral hygiene if it didn't remind you of dessert?

Finally, FD&C Blue 1 and Red 40 are used to dye toothpaste (mouthwash, too)—but they come with dangers. According to the Center for Science in the Public Interest (CSPI), Red 40 poses "risks including hyperactivity and other behavior problems in children." In Europe, products containing these dyes must carry a warning label; one study found Red 40 that was contaminated with the carcinogen benzidine, a chemical used in the dye's production. CSPI also warned that Blue No. 1 has the potential to cause neurotoxicity and cautions against its use by children (although it can be found in children's toothpaste).

And then, in addition to all that stuff, there's fluoride—a chemical with a past.

Early in the twentieth century, scientists discovered that areas with high levels of naturally occurring fluoride in their drinking water also had low levels of tooth decay. In 1945, Grand Rapids, Michigan, became the first city in the world to add the chemical to its tap water. Children there began having fewer cavities, and soon the practice spread throughout the country—to the point where the CDC praised fluoridation as one of the "ten great public health achievements" of the twentieth century. Effortlessly, American children would enjoy great dental health for the rest of their lives.

Even back then, however, experts worried about possible harmful effects of drinking so much fluoride. But those concerns were dismissed—for a while. Because once fluoride's benefits for tooth health became known, toothpaste manufacturers started including it in their products, meaning that kids and everyone else got even more of the chemical. Then researchers looking into fluoride's side effects began reporting some alarming results.

The main danger of fluoride has to do with its toxic effects on developing brains. According to a 2012 report from the Harvard T. H. Chan School of Public Health, "Children in high-fluoride areas had significantly lower IQ scores than those who lived in low-fluoride areas."

And the National Research Council (NRC) of the National Academy of Sciences has raised concerns about links between fluoride and bone cancer, bone fractures, and reproductive system problems.

Clearly, fluoride's reputation has taken a beating since local governments began adding it to everyone's tap water. Take a look at what the FDA now requires toothpaste manufacturers to include on the label for products containing fluoride:

> WARNING: Keep out of reach of children under 6 years of age. If more than used for brushing is accidentally swallowed, get medical help or contact a Poison Control Center right away.

As a result of that warning, there are now more than twenty thousand reports each year to poison control centers in the United States due to excessive ingestion of fluoride toothpaste.

It's important to keep in mind that the problems with fluoride stem from drinking it—not brushing your teeth with products containing it. It remains true that using a fluoride toothpaste benefits children's teeth (adults' teeth, not so much).

It's possible to give your kids beautiful, healthy, cavity-free smiles without subtracting from their IQs. Just be sure to tell them: Don't swallow! And maybe if you stick with brands that don't taste as minty and sweet as candy, they won't.

Dental Floss

We have to thank Levi Parmly (1790–1859), widely recognized as the father of dental hygiene, for most of the oral health practices we follow today, especially flossing. He recognized that cavities were caused by food that got stuck between the teeth that brushing couldn't remove. So in 1815, he began promoting the use of waxed silk thread as "the most important" tool to prevent tooth decay. According to Mary Duenwald in the *New York Times*:

[Parmly] was not above proselytizing on the street. "If he noticed that someone's mouth was not in a good state of repair, he would buttonhole him," said Dr. Arden G. Christen, who teaches dental history at Indiana University. Parmly would hand out floss and teach people how to use it.

That must have been quite a sight!

Like brushing, flossing is necessary if we want to have a healthy mouth. But manufacturers have added unnecessary, potentially harmful ingredients, so we need to be cautious.

Old-school floss, for all its benefits, had a downside—all that sawing back and forth between the teeth hurts and makes our gums bleed. An early fix was to coat it in wax, causing it to move more easily. Then, because corporate innovation never rests, somebody came up with floss that is wide and flat like a ribbon instead of thin and round like string. On top of that, a Teflon-like chemical was used to coat the floss to allow it to slide through the spaces between teeth without any friction at all.

It was a genius move, except for one little detail: the coating was made from the PFAS family of "forever chemicals," which pop up time and again in the world of Fatal Conveniences. These are the substances that almost all of us have ingested one way or another and have been linked to cancer, liver damage, cognitive developmental issues, and a long list of other serious health problems.

Are there PFASs in your brand of floss? It's hard to say, because floss is considered a medical device and so there are no labeling requirements. But a study of women who used one popular brand of friction-free floss found PFAS chemicals in their blood. Scary.

In addition to floss being slippery, it's also now flavored, usually with mint, the universal symbol of wonderful breath. What exactly is in that flavoring? That's a good question, but we'll never know, for the same reason we don't know anything else about floss: it's considered to be a medical device and thus is exempt from the FDA's labeling rules.

Does all this mean that flossing your teeth can cause cancer? Who knows? Once a day you're putting a chemical linked to cancer and other diseases into contact with your delicate mouth tissues. Doesn't sound like the smartest thing in the world, does it?

As I've said, there are way too many hazardous and carcinogenic chemicals already inside our bodies, due just to living on this planet at this moment in time. Why add to the toxic load if we don't have to? To me, that's a good reason to stick with old-school, mildly painful floss that does more good than harm.

Mouthwash

Finally, we come to the iffiest oral hygiene product: mouthwash.

There are references to mouth rinsing in Chinese medicine circa 2700 BCE and in the ancient Greek and Roman periods, too. The rinses typically contained salt, alum, vinegar, and maybe some anise. Later versions used wine or beer.

But mouthwash as we know it was developed in the late 1800s, and it usually contained alcohol. In 1879, a product you may have heard of— Listerine—was introduced as an antiseptic for use in surgery and for sterilizing wounds. By 1914, however, it had been repurposed as a mouthwash due to its effectiveness at killing germs.

In 1920, the makers of Listerine came up with a game changer: they took an obscure, minor medical condition, halitosis, and used their marketing muscle to turn it into a twentieth-century anxiety. Suddenly, what had been a mere social liability (and probably an extremely common one) became a treatable ailment, and sales of the medicinal-tasting stuff took off.

Which is not to say that bad breath doesn't exist, because it sure does, as we're all painfully aware. There are many possible causes, including:

+ Bacteria buildup on the teeth (in which case you need to brush and floss more)
+ Gum disease

+ Improperly cleaned dentures
+ Infections of the nose, windpipe, or lungs
+ A condition called xerostomia, or dry mouth. Because of low saliva production, the mouth can't cleanse itself by carrying away leftover bits of food and other debris. It may also be caused by certain medicines, a salivary gland disorder, or breathing through the mouth instead of the nose.
+ Chronic bronchitis
+ Postnasal drip
+ Chronic sinusitis
+ Diabetes
+ Disorders of the liver, kidneys, or gastrointestinal system

Or you might just have eaten garlic or onions, smoked cigarettes, or ingested other things that will make your breath stink no matter how many oral care products you use.

Mouthwash is overrated and exists mainly to treat insecurity, not halitosis. There's actually a psychological condition called *halitophobia*, the unfounded fear that you have bad breath. Unless you have lousy oral hygiene or a treatable medical problem, your breath probably smells no worse than anyone else's.

In fact, there's research showing that mouthwash could actually be causing health problems. One study found that using it twice a day was associated with an increased risk of prediabetes or diabetes, while rinsing less than twice a day had no such effect. Why might this be so? Researchers speculate it's because the antibacterials in mouthwash kill off the good microbes with the bad—and the lack of "good" actinobacteria is thought to raise nitrate levels in the blood and increase the risk of developing type 2 diabetes.

Another study found that mouthwash containing chlorhexidine, when used twice a day for a week, increased the amount of certain bacteria and created an environment that's favorable for cavities (and is also possibly detrimental to cardiovascular health). Also, although chlorhexidine is used in mouthwash to control plaque and gingivitis, researchers in Italy found that it can stain teeth and tongue. That's not exactly what we're going for when we obsess over our oral grooming.

Okay, So What Should We Do?

There are lots of ways to minimize the downside of modern oral hygiene practices. First, consume mainly whole plants, fruits, nuts, seeds, legumes, and natural herbs and spices. These all have a natural cleansing effect rather than fouling your mouth and body with ultraprocessed garbage. You can chew on rosemary, spearmint, or peppermint leaves for that fresh, minty taste. Frankincense, myrrh, and white oak bark all have antiseptic and anti-inflammatory properties, and chewing them is a great way to support healthy gums and rebuild enamel. Finally, drinking a glass of water with lemon juice in the morning knocks out overnight bacteria.

Here's another good idea: don't pay attention to social media ads or TV commercials. The actors in them squeeze enough toothpaste onto one brush for an entire family. The reason this is done is obvious: if you do the same, you'll go through a tube about twice as fast as necessary.

If the idea of consuming fluoride makes you uncomfortable, there are nontoxic alternatives, including plant extracts such as pomegranate, garlic, and ginger. Some popular natural toothpaste makers use xylitol, green tea extract, papaya plant extract, and baking soda. If you've been eating something odiferous, sucking sugar-free mints or chewing gum might do the trick. And if you're sick and tired of flossing, try a rechargeable electric flosser, which shoots a stream of water between your teeth to dislodge anything that might be stuck there.

FATAL CONVENIENCE: FRAGRANCE

What's so bad about smelling good?

It's no mystery why the world of consumer products is obsessed with fragrances. To a huge degree, our behaviors are driven by our olfactory sense, whether we're talking about food, flowers, new car interiors, or bubble bath—or other people. Our emotions are powerfully triggered by scent, and we're pretty much helpless to resist the lure.

This is why manufacturers add fragrance to just about everything you buy. It's ubiquitous in the personal care category, though it's also present everywhere else—you didn't believe corn chips or T-shirts smell that way naturally, did you? Clearly, we need to be on the lookout, but what exactly are we looking for? As I've already said, it's impossible to know which substances are used to make products smell good. On the label, all you're likely to see is "fragrance" or "parfum," and you can guess why manufacturers obscure an iffy ingredient.

The chemical groups found most often in fragrances are benzenoids, terpenes, and musks. All of these are found in nature, which doesn't necessarily mean they're nontoxic. At any rate, the ones used in fragrance are all made using industrial processes. Even musk, which was originally sourced from a gland found next to a musk deer's penis, is now mostly man-made (because it's cheaper, not out of any regard for the musk deer's feelings).

Whether natural or synthesized, commercial scents are irritating to many people, who experience allergic reactions whether they are worn by others or themselves. A 2020 study found that up to 4.5 percent of people may be allergic to fragrance chemicals used most often in deodorants, perfumes, and aftershaves. Another study found that over one-third of Americans suffer adverse health effects, such as respiratory difficulties and migraine headaches, from exposure to fragranced products. That's because even "natural" chemicals emit gases known as volatile organic compounds, or VOCs. No wonder people who overdo it with cologne are shunned as walking irritants.

But allergic reactions are the least of our worries.

Throughout this book we've seen warnings about the chemicals known as phthalates. They're added to fragrance products to make the scent last longer. According to the FDA, a common one, diethylphthalate, or DEP, "does not pose known risks for human health as it is currently used in cosmetics and fragrances." But a 2022 study found that exposure to this chemical and other phthalates is associated with cardiovascular and all-cause mortality. Previous research had linked the chemicals to increases in premature births, gestational diabetes, obesity, breast and thyroid cancers, and infertility. They are also "among the most abundant endocrine disrupting compounds found in indoor air and dust," according to researchers from the Albert Einstein College of Medicine, who added that exposure to phthalates can affect bone mineral density and sperm function.

Aldehydes are found naturally in plants and are used as fragrance enhancers—they're what give Chanel No. 5 its legendary scent. One type of aldehyde, acetaldehyde, is found in ripe fruit and is used to add a fruity fragrance. But the International Agency for Research on Cancer considers it a carcinogen, and it's included on California's Proposition 65 list of cancer warnings. Can we know for sure that it's in the fragrances we wear? No, but a study from the 1980s found that exposure to sunlight affects the compounds in perfume bottles, turning ethanol into acetaldehyde.

Fragrance ingredients carry the same danger of hormone disruption as in other personal care product chemicals. A German study published in 2002 found that women with premenstrual symptoms and infertility had higher levels of artificial musk in their blood samples than women who had been pregnant already and didn't have premenstrual syndrome. Researchers from the Albert Einstein College of Medicine in New York City have warned that "health concerns associated with exposures to synthetic musks include primarily endocrine disruption."

How About the Environment?

There are data indicating that synthetic musk fragrance compounds are found in high concentrations in fresh water and the fish that live there, suggesting that these chemicals persist long after they go down the drain. A study in China found that synthetic musks were found in high concentrations in the muscle tissues of fish and shrimp in a lake, and they've been found in Lake Michigan as well. Additional research from Stanford University's Hopkins Marine Station found that musks "inhibited natural defenses against toxicants in California mussels, and that the effect remained long after exposure."

Finally, a 2021 study found that emissions from fragranced personal care and cleaning products account for at least *half* of the ozone attributed to volatile chemical products in Manhattan! The environment's going to hell, but gee, don't we smell great?

Okay, So What Should We Do?

Here's the best advice I can offer: don't use any product that lists "fragrance" or "parfum" on the ingredients label. If the manufacturer doesn't tell you exactly what's in the product, it must have a reason, and it's probably not a good one. Even better, try to avoid products that contain fragrance; look for those labeled "fragrance free." Believe me, as long as you and your clothes are clean, you already smell good enough. You don't need some industrial lab concoction to make you more lovable than you already are. If wearing fragrance is important to you, try using one of the many essential oils or other all-natural substances that people perfumed themselves with for centuries before big business took over. Beyond that:

+ Look for labels saying that products are phthalate free.
+ Insist on ingredient transparency. Even though they're not required to list fragrance ingredients, some companies now volunteer this information. L'Oréal announced in 2021 that it will be disclosing ingredients on its products and on its website. Unilever now reveals its products' ingredients as well. Procter & Gamble is disclosing fragrance components online via SmartLabel (smartlabel.org) and its website. It even includes a list of ingredients it *doesn't* use. Johnson & Johnson has committed to fragrance transparency, but as of this writing, only for baby products. Tom's of Maine backs up its claims of using only naturally sourced or derived materials for its products

by listing ingredients to the 100 parts per million in its fragrance ingredients disclosure info.

+ Check for the EPA Safer Choice label. It means a company is committed to using fragrances without "listed carcinogens, mutagens, or reproductive/developmental toxicants (CMRs); listed persistent, bioaccumulative, and toxic compounds (PBTs); and listed respiratory sensitizers." You can search for certified products on the agency's website (epa.gov).

FATAL CONVENIENCE: SUNSCREEN

There's something weird about the fact that although the sun is the source of all life on our planet, we've been taught to fear it. Without the light and heat of that big star 93 million miles away, we wouldn't exist, and neither would plants or anything else we eat.

Among all the other wonderful things sunlight gives us is the amazing ability to create, within our bodies, vitamin D, which keeps us alive and healthy by regulating at least a thousand different genes, including those involved in immune system function. It even protects us from cancer.

Vitamin D production isn't the only blessing that comes with exposure to sunlight. We evolved to be outdoors when the sun shines and asleep when it's dark. That's why our pineal glands synthesize melatonin at night, to help us sleep soundly. There's research showing that catching rays turns on beneficial neural pathways, and even artificial light in the morning promotes better sleep the next night and is effective against PMS and seasonal affective disorder, or SAD, the depression some people experience during the gray and gloomy months of the year.

Why are we so afraid of the sun? Number one, because we've been told over and over about the risk of skin cancer from exposure to the sun's ultraviolet rays, a legitimate worry. There's also a cosmetic reason: the idea that our skin will age more quickly and wrinkle if we get too much direct sunlight. It's hard to tell which of those two we fear most, but we've been indoctrinated with the fairly recent idea that we need to hide from the sun.

Which is how sunscreen came to be practically a requirement today—even though these creams and lotions come with their own health hazards, which may be more dangerous than what we're using them to protect us from.

The American Academy of Dermatology says we should wear sunscreen every time we step outdoors, even on the cloudiest winter days. It also says, "Claims that any of these ingredients are toxic or a hazard to human health have not been proven."

That isn't exactly true.

In fact, according to the FDA, of all the active ingredients found in sunscreens, only two are "generally recognized as safe and effective": zinc oxide and titanium dioxide, both natural substances.

There's a much longer roster of chemicals still in use that the FDA decided *not* to put on its "safe and effective" list. You may already be aware of one of them—by now many people avoid using sunscreen containing para-aminobenzoic acid, or PABA. Also on the FDA list: trolamine salicylate, cinoxate, dioxybenzone, ensulizole, homosalate, meradimate, octinoxate, octisalate, octocrylene, padimate O, sulisobenzone, oxybenzone, and avobenzone. The FDA usually lags behind the rest of the scientific world in recognizing industrial chemicals as being health hazards, so when it worries a little about a substance, we should worry a lot.

The European Commission says that some of the chemicals on that list are unsafe in the amounts currently used in sunscreen and has recommended drastic cuts in the levels allowed. Meanwhile, US manufacturers are legally permitted to use those chemicals at even higher levels—far exceeding what Europe will tolerate for its citizens. For example, after a single application of sunscreen, subjects' blood concentrations of oxybenzone were more than 180 times the FDA's level of concern. They soared to *more than five hundred times* the FDA's own threshold after four days' use as recommended on the label!

According to studies published by the FDA, six of the chemicals used in sunscreen are absorbed into the body after just one use and can still be detected on the skin and in the blood weeks after being applied. All the chemicals on that list are suspected or proven endocrine disruptors. High levels of oxybenzone found in the blood of adolescent boys resulted in significantly lower testosterone levels. The chemical has also been associated with shorter pregnancies, lower birth weights, and increased risk of developing breast cancer and endometriosis. It's also possible that because it is an anti-inflammatory, it might actually hide the symptoms of sunburn and keep it from being treated.

There's even the potential for danger from a known carcinogen that is *not* listed among sunscreen ingredients. Research conducted by an independent lab found benzene in 27 percent of the sunscreen samples they tested, including the most popular brands. A 2021 study found yet another dangerous chemical that isn't on the ingredients list: octocrylene. When this degrades, it can turn into benzophenone, also an endocrine disruptor and carcinogen.

The fact is that most of us are flying blind when it comes to sunscreen. We assume that choosing the highest SPF we can find is the way to go, but that's no guarantee of safety or anything else. The EWG found that 85 percent of sunscreen products with an SPF rating of 15 or higher provide inadequate protection from UV rays or have ingredients that either are known health hazards or have not been tested for safety. Nearly every sunscreen from leading brands failed to meet EWG's standards for safety and effectiveness. Some studies suggest that sunscreen with SPF 30 or higher reduces vitamin D production in the body by a whopping 95 to 98 percent—kind of counterproductive, considering that vitamin D helps protect us from cancer. You are being told to protect yourself from overexposure to the sun and cancer by using sunscreen when some of its ingredients can potentially cause cancer or drastically reduce your body's ability to protect against it!

Does that make sense?

How About the Environment?

Two of the chemicals found in sunscreen, oxybenzone and octinox-ate, have been banned by the state of Hawaii and the city of Key West, Florida, because they threaten the health of the marine ecosystem. Knowing that, ask yourself: Do they belong on your skin and in your bloodstream?

Okay, So What Should We Do?

The first thing we should do is make sure we're soaking up enough direct sunlight for our health. Vitamin D researchers recommend half an hour of exposure between 10:00 a.m. and 3:00 p.m. at least twice a week to the face, arms, legs, or back—*without* sunscreen. Make sure to factor in your existing tan. The lighter you are, the less time you need in the sun.

If you're worried about getting too much sun on your face, wear a nontoxic sunscreen (and maybe a hat). But weather permitting, make sure your arms and legs are bare, so you absorb enough UV to guarantee your supply of vitamin D. If for some reason you can't get out in the sun—or if you live where there's not much sunlight during winter months—the moderate use of commercial tanning beds that emit 2 to 6 percent UVB radiation is considered a safe and effective way to supplement vitamin D.

We should also recognize that we don't need *any* lotion to protect us from the sun; we can just cover up or go inside during the hottest part of the day. Even the World Health Organization advises us to first try limiting our exposure to direct sunlight *before* automatically applying sunscreen. On most weather apps you can check the UV index and plan your outdoor time accordingly. Finally, eating foods high in antioxidants will protect your skin, along with the rest of your body, from the effects of too much sun exposure.

What *is* important is to avoid getting sunburned, since bad burns are believed to be the cause of skin cancers later in life.

We need to keep in mind that although skin cancer is the most common form of the disease, melanoma, the kind that kills, was responsible for just 1.2 percent of all cancer deaths in 2021. Despite what the American Academy of Dermatology tells us, there's no one-size-fits-all advice when it comes to sunlight exposure and cancer. Your skin color, for instance, is a factor: lighter-skinned people need to be more careful about spending too much time in direct sunlight. Statistically, the lifetime risk of developing melanoma is 2.6 percent (1 in 38) for whites, 0.6 percent (1 in 167) for Hispanics, and 0.1 percent (1 in 1,000) for Blacks.

One special category is children, for the simple reason that adult melanoma is believed to be a result of bad sunburns that occur in childhood. It takes that long for the cancer to develop. So one way or another, they need to be protected through common sense, though it's best to do so by limiting their exposure to sunlight rather than coating them in sketchy chemicals.

As I already said, when it's absolutely necessary, go with sunscreens containing zinc oxide or titanium dioxide. Unlike all the other kinds, which contain a chemical filter, these two create a physical barrier that absorbs sunlight before it reaches your skin. That's why they're thicker and harder to apply, which is a little inconvenient, I agree. But they're a lot safer in the long run.

Finally, stick with sunscreen lotions—the spray-on kind doesn't protect us adequately from the sun's rays.

In the end, there's a proper balance we need to strike, Goldilocks style, between getting enough sunlight to produce vitamin D and getting too much and risking skin cancer. It's possible to find that sweet spot if we try.

FATAL CONVENIENCES: TAMPONS

When you consider all the substances women have used to absorb menstrual blood—grass, wool, paper, sponge—it's easy to see why tampons were a godsend. The fact that they could be inserted into the body, rather than worn on the outside like cumbersome pads, makes them really appealing. Today, an estimated 70 percent of American women who menstruate use tampons, meaning that by now they are no longer mere conveniences—they're necessities.

The fact that they're regulated by the FDA as medical devices should be reassuring. But as we've seen elsewhere, a federal agency's oversight doesn't always mean we're being protected. Tampons and other menstrual products, including pads, can contain phthalates due to the fragrances that some brands add. They might also include parabens, bisphenol A, and triclocarban, endocrine disruptors that can cause:

+ Endometriosis
+ Ovulation disorders
+ Hormonal disorders
+ Allergic reactions

Tampons may contain dioxins, the chemical by-product of converting wood pulp into rayon, the absorbent fabric that is often used. The EPA says that high levels of dioxins put us at risk of developing:

+ Immune system damage
+ Increased risk of pelvic inflammatory disease
+ Reduced fertility

According to the FDA, dioxin exposure from tampons "is many times less than normally present in the body from other environmental sources." That might be so, but it's still concerning for two reasons: the mucous membranes lining the vagina are permeable and connect to the ovaries and uterus; and dioxins may cause cancer. The fact that we're taking in even more dioxins from other sources in the environment isn't reassuring—just the opposite. Because vaginal skin is so thin, researchers also estimate that endocrine-disrupting chemicals from menstrual products are absorbed at a rate ten times as high as elsewhere on the body.

In addition to the dangers from their chemical contents, tampons pose another threat, which made headlines back in the 1980s: reports of women getting sick and even dying from toxic shock syndrome, or TSS, a multisystem infection caused by leaving tampons in for too long. That was the result of yet another "convenience"; a new innovation, "maximum absorbency tampons," was leading users to replace them less frequently. The synthetic contents that caused toxic shock are no longer used. But the risk of infection from tampons will always remain.

How About the Environment?

Globally, an estimated 7 billion tampons are used every year. Like diapers, they're made with absorbent synthetic materials that don't decompose in a hurry. Over the forty or so years during which the average woman menstruates, the estimated sixteen thousand tampons (and applicators) she uses will end up in landfills or even in our waterways. Throw in another four hundred pounds of packaging on top of that.

Okay, So What Should We Do?

Look for brands that are unbleached, fragrance free, and made without dyes or hydrogen peroxide (used for whitening).

Use brands made with organic cotton.

Use tampons without plastic applicators.

Change tampons every four hours to prevent toxic shock syndrome.

Try menstrual products from companies committed to using healthy, all-natural ingredients, like organic cotton.

Consider giving up tampons altogether! One alternative is the menstrual cup, from brands such as Nixit, DivaCup, and Cora. Hesitant to make the switch? A study done in Vancouver found that 91 percent of tampon users said they'd switch after trying a cup. You want medical-grade silicone, BPA free, of course.

Another choice is reusable pads, from companies including Hannah,

Tree Hugger, and New Moon, or period underwear from Thinx, Knix, or TomboyX.

Finally, there is a movement to force manufacturers to list all ingredients used in tampons. Find a petition online and sign it!

FATAL CONVENIENCE: LIPSTICK

There are two factors peculiar to lipstick and lip gloss that should make wearers worry. Number one is that the skin on our lips is much thinner than that pretty much anywhere else on our bodies. That thinness means we absorb whatever we put onto our lips. Number two is that lipstick wearers can't help swallowing some of it. They have it on from morning until bedtime and apply it several times during a normal day. You're constantly wetting your lips with your tongue—we all do. And every time, a little bit of lipstick stays on your tongue, slides down your throat, and enters your stomach, where it is absorbed into your tissues just like anything else you eat or drink. Not a lot, but some.

There's a third thing, too: lead. There are also other dangerous metals, including chromium, cadmium, aluminum, and manganese, all of which are contained in the pigment. Lead, as you probably know, is a neurotoxin. It builds up in the body and damages the brain. It's why when children are exposed to lead in paint or drinking water, the results are so devastating. They suffer from learning, language, and behavioral disorders. Exposure to lead has also been linked to other health concerns, among them:

+ Reduced fertility in both men and women
+ Hormonal changes and menstrual irregularities
+ Delayed onset of puberty

In 2007, the Campaign for Safe Cosmetics released a report titled *A Poison Kiss*, for which an independent laboratory tested thirty-three popular brands of lipsticks for lead content. It found that 61 percent of lipsticks, including those made by the biggest names in the business, tested positive for the metal. The FDA and cosmetics companies insist that the metals in lipsticks occur at such low levels that they pose no harm. But according to the CDC, there is *no such thing* as a safe level of lead—for anyone. In addition, according to a CDC fact sheet, "Pregnant women and women of childbearing age should avoid exposure to lead because lead ingested by a mother can affect the unborn child."

We all ought to be extra careful about what we wear on our lips. And lipstick makers should be extra cautious, knowing that their customers will be not only wearing their product but eating it.

Heavy metals aren't the only dangerous thing about lipstick. It also contains a category of industrial chemicals called D4 and D5, which we find everywhere in cosmetics and personal care products. They are bio-accumulative, meaning that they build up in our bodies and also in the environment once we wash the makeup off and it goes down the drain and into the waterways. The Canadian government has declared these chemicals toxic, and the European Union placed them on its restricted substances list because they are endocrine disruptors.

Okay, So What Should We Do?

Do you want to be 100 percent sure you aren't exposing your lips, mouth, and body to the harmful ingredients in lipstick? Don't wear it! I know, I know that's probably not realistic. But maybe you can wear less. Or use a brand made with nontoxic ingredients. Here's a list of some of the natural substances that health-conscious companies put into safe lip products:

+ Elderberry extract
+ Moringa oil
+ Organic avocado oil
+ Organic plum seed oil
+ Organic hemp seed oil
+ Organic neem oil

- Organic orange oil
- Sunflower seed wax
- Soy butter
- Kokum butter
- Candelilla wax
- Beet powder

They sound a lot safer than the industrial chemicals found in conventional cosmetics, don't they?

Here are some companies to try for safer lip products.

- Axiology, which proclaims that none of its cosmetics contains more than ten ingredients, and they're vegan and cruelty free with no palm oil
- Hourglass, a great vegan brand
- Lush, vegan lipstick containing broccoli seeds!
- Kuwaloo, a small, eco-friendly UK-based brand making handmade mineral lip and cheek balm
- Inika, the world's first certified organic vegan range of lipsticks
- E.L.F., Smashbox, and Kylie Cosmetics, vegan brands
- Honest Beauty
- Boomstick Glo

FATAL CONVENIENCE: SHAVING CREAM

On the face of it—no pun intended, honest—shaving should be simple. There's your skin, your blade, and a substance to go between the two to protect you from cuts and irritations and make the process work smoothly. Whatever product you use is in place for a few moments only. No sooner do you put it on than you remove it.

We're not content to keep things so basic, of course. Way back in the 1970s, Joe Namath and Farrah Fawcett made shaving cream sexy, at least if you believed their TV commercial. There was also the one where the gorgeous Swedish model cooed, "Take it off . . . take it all off." (She was referring to shaving cream, wasn't she?) Suddenly, the boring daily task of removing stubble became a whole lot more interesting than when our prehistoric ancestors scraped their cheeks with flint, clam shells, or pieces of bronze.

For the most part, the active ingredients in shaving products aren't toxic: nearly 80 percent water, plus something to remove your skin's natural lubricant so the whiskers are easier to cut, plus something else to moisturize and soothe the skin. But those aren't the only substances present.

As I've mentioned before, the "forever chemicals" known as PFASs, PFOAs, and PFC are found in thousands of products we use every day. Their main job is to make things slippery, as in Teflon nonstick cooking surfaces, but they are also present in shaving cream. They make your skin sleek and smooth, which sounds like a nice idea until you remember that these chemicals have been linked to several kinds of cancer (including testicular), thyroid problems, high cholesterol levels, colitis, and more.

They have also been linked to developmental and hormonal dysfunction in children and abnormal fetal development in pregnant women (including a possible higher incidence of infant death). As if all that weren't bad enough, the chemicals are persistent, meaning that they accumulate in both our bodies and the environment. These substances are dangerous—definitely not the kind of thing you want to slap onto your face every morning or use to shave your legs. You're already being exposed to these chemicals in so many ways, why add one more?

Triethanolamine is another common ingredient, used to soften skin and adjust the pH of shaving cream. It's not classified as cancer causing, but the National Cancer Institute has studied it due to concerns that it can turn into the carcinogen N-nitrosodiethanolamine. Polyethylene glycol (PEG), a chemical that acts as a thickener and emulsifier, is found in many personal care products, including shaving cream. It's not hazardous—except for the fact that contaminants frequently found in PEG, 1,4-dioxane and ethylene oxide, which are part of the manufacturing process and often present as impurities, are *both* carcinogenic. This is a good reminder that not every ingredient in any product, even food, is listed on the label. Sometimes the offending substances are in the product unintentionally and anonymously—which doesn't make them any less lethal.

A big part of shaving cream's appeal is the way it smells: clean and soapy. But the manufacturers won't tell us exactly which chemicals they use to create those scents, so we're better off skipping anything with the word *fragrance* or *parfum* on the label.

How About the Environment?

Shaving cream's harm to the environment comes not so much from the product itself but from the delivery method. First, there's the metal can. According to the EPA, in one year around 3.75 billion aerosol cans (of all products, not just shaving cream) are filled in the United States alone. That in itself is a huge environmental burden, in both the making and the disposing—especially for a product that doesn't really need such a heavy-duty container. The other hazard is the propellant. Until the 1970s, ozone-depleting chlorofluorocarbons (CFCs) were the main propellant used in aerosol cans. Today manufacturers use hydrocarbons or compressed gas, which is an improvement, but these still give off volatile organic compounds, which damage the environment and aren't so great for us, either.

Okay, So What Should We Do?

You could just give up shaving cream altogether, because it's unnecessary. Instead, apply whatever bodywash or soap you use on the rest of your skin, preferably one without harmful chemicals. Women have the right idea: they lather up and shave in the shower. That's a little difficult for a man to do, unless you have a nonfogging mirror in there. But it's possible.

Or do what I do: use a little organic coconut oil, which will lubricate your skin so the razor can do its job without causing irritation. I sometimes shave in the shower with chemical-free soap. I haven't used shaving cream since I was eighteen years old! Who needs it?

If you feel the need to use a shaving product, pick a soap or cream with as few ingredients as you can find and without any of the garbage I've discussed in this chapter. Pay attention to the packaging, and definitely do not use anything that comes in an aerosol spray can.

You could also try an electric razor. Or grow a beard.

FATAL CONVENIENCE: DEODORANT

The ability to sweat is one of the countless miracles responsible for our continued presence on this planet. But not everybody loves it. And—as happens so often—our attempts to outsmart Mother Nature only bring us to grief.

Perspiration is our built-in air-conditioning system, designed to keep us at a proper body temperature even when, due to exertion or external temperatures, we're overheating. If we couldn't sweat, we'd bake inside our skins like potatoes and then die. Along with our livers and kidneys, perspiration rids our bodies of waste.

Sweat is around 99 percent water, along with urea, uric acid, ammonia, lactic acid, vitamin C, and some other stuff. But it's not the perspiration itself that causes body odor; that arises when it mixes with the bacteria on our skin. Since we have so many sweat glands under our arms, where it's warm and dark, they're a natural hot spot of stink.

Once upon a time, when bathing habits were more relaxed, either you masked your body odor with perfume or you lived with it, the same as everybody around you. People were more pungent back then, no doubt, but probably less insecure when it came to social acceptability.

Then, in 1888, an inventor came up with Mum, a cream containing an antibacterial, zinc oxide. It didn't stop you from sweating, but it took away the smell. And in 1903, there was a fateful step forward: a product called Everdry used aluminum salts to prevent sweat from even forming, an innovation that probably seemed brilliant—at the time.

Now we know that the deodorant-related danger comes from precisely that feature. Under various names (aluminum chlorohydrate, aluminum zirconium tetrachlorohydrex, aluminum zirconium trichlorohydrex), it is the key ingredient in all antiperspirant deodorants: the metal ions mix with sugar molecules in the sweat to form plugs that obstruct the sweat glands and stop sweat from escaping. Because we have these glands all over our bodies, the perspiration just comes out elsewhere, so we don't overheat.

Deodorant keeps our armpits arid, but what else does it do?

Aluminum has been linked to cancer, especially of the breast tissue due to the armpit's proximity. Research suggests that the metal salts cause changes in the estrogen receptors of breast cells, thereby increasing the risk of the disease. When Austrian researchers asked around four hundred women about their use of antiperspirants before the age of thirty, it was discovered that those who had applied it several times a day were more likely to have aluminum in their breast tissue—and also more likely to develop breast cancer.

According to a 2005 paper in the *Journal of Inorganic Biochemistry*:

> Clinical studies showing a disproportionately high incidence of breast cancer in the upper outer quadrant of the breast together with reports of genomic instability in outer quadrants of the breast provide supporting evidence for a role for locally applied cosmetic chemicals in the development of breast cancer. Aluminum is known to have a genotoxic profile, capable of causing both DNA alterations and epigenetic effects, and this would be consistent with a potential role in breast cancer if such effects occurred in breast cells.

The American Cancer Society says there is no clear link between antiperspirants and breast cancer because no epidemiological studies have confirmed the connection. Other research, according to the ACS, has found that breast cancer tissue doesn't contain any more aluminum than healthy tissue.

So there's no smoking-gun proof that aluminum in deodorant can cause cancer. On the other hand, there are plenty of hints that point in that direction. I say: when in doubt, leave it out. There's no possible advantage to having dry armpits that's worth the risk of breast cancer (and remember that men get breast cancer, too).

There could also be a link between aluminum and Alzheimer's disease. A study from the 1980s found that people with the ailment had accumulations of aluminum in their brain neurons. (To be fair, the experts say it may have gotten there through contaminated water, food, or medications.)

Some deodorants also contain polypropylene glycol, which can irritate the skin but is considered otherwise harmless. It should come as no surprise that big-brand products contain all the poisonous stuff we find everywhere in the personal care aisles: parabens, fragrance, triclosan, phthalates, and benzene in aerosol sprays. Sprays, with their hydrocarbons, are particularly harmful. By now I hope I don't have to warn you: stay away from this junk.

Finally, we've all heard about the importance of the microbiome, the bacteria in our gut that determine our health in a multitude of ways. Your skin has its own microbiome, and there's a study suggesting that antiperspirants kill it off—one more way this personal care product harms rather than helps us.

How About the Environment?

Even if you aren't concerned about the potential health hazards of antiperspirants, the environmental impact might worry you: though aluminum occurs naturally in the environment, humans have increased the concentration of it in drinking water. This is a problem not only for us but for other animals because aluminum acts as a neurotoxin, affecting the motor and cognitive abilities of aquatic vertebrates such as frogs. There's also all that plastic in containers and packaging that we're adding to the global overload.

Okay, So What Should We Do?

First, try to cut back on your deodorant use. Go without it one day, and see if you (or anyone else) notices the difference. It's possible that you've been worrying about nothing all these years.

Use brands with as few ingredients as you can find.

Some deodorants use talc to absorb moisture, but that can be contaminated with asbestos, a carcinogen. Try brands with cornstarch or tapioca starch instead. They are naturally zero aluminum.

And don't use aerosol sprays—in anything, not just deodorant, due to the benzene they contain. Use stick or roll-on products.

Believe it or not, botulinum toxin, popularly known as botox, has been approved to eliminate underarm sweating. When injected, it blocks the signals that tell our glands it's time to perspire. Originally, it was used to treat people afflicted with overactive sweat glands on the hands, then to paralyze facial muscles and give people a more youthful appearance. Underarms need about twenty-five shots each and cost around $2,000 per treatment, which is only temporary. That sounds slightly insane to me, but it has the advantage of not introducing any harmful chemicals into our bodies.

FATAL CONVENIENCE: EYE MAKEUP

From Queen Nefertiti and Cleopatra thousands of years ago to Rihanna and Kim Kardashian today, bold black eye makeup has knocked us out with its beauty. At various times in history—even recent history—men, too, have sported eyeliner and mascara. Hello, Johnny Depp!

In ancient times it was made of kohl, a mineral that might actually have had some antibacterial powers (not a small consideration before antibiotics came along). But kohl also contains antimony, lead, and other dangerous heavy metals, and when you apply it to the ultrathin skin surrounding the eyes, you're asking for trouble. For that reason, it's banned from cosmetic use today.

What has replaced it? Parabens, propylene glycol, phthalates, petroleum—in other words, more toxic and even carcinogenic substances, the same ones that show up in so many other personal care products today. The fact that these are worn so close to the eyes poses the same dangers as kohl did, so maybe we haven't really spared ourselves much harm.

Realistically, how much of the harmful contents of eye makeup do we absorb? That question was answered in a 2016 study conducted by Dr. Kim Harley, a reproductive epidemiologist at the University of California, Berkeley. First, she tested the urine of a hundred adolescent girls who used conventional makeup and found detectable levels of phthalates and parabens—both of which are potentially endocrine-disrupting chemicals, meaning they can alter sex hormones. For the next three days, the girls used makeup that contained none of those substances, and their urine was tested again—and the levels of both chemicals had already fallen, "by 25 to 45 percent, on average," Harley said. A huge reduction!

Okay, So What Should We Do?

One alternative is to wear less eye makeup. We don't always need to look as though we're ready to be swarmed by paparazzi or headed to a glamorous night on the red carpet. We can give our eyes a break once in a while. Young women, whose hormones don't need any extra interference, should be especially cautious when choosing eye makeup. Read the tiny print on the label and beware of the following ingredients.

+ Carbon black, sometimes called D&C Black No. 2, acetylene black, or channel black
+ Ethanolamine compounds, which are used as emulsifiers and fragrances and are potentially carcinogenic. On labels, they're called triethanolamine (TEA), diethanolamine (DEA), cocamide DEA, cocamide MEA, DEA-cetyl phosphate, DEA-oleth-3 phosphate, lauramide DEA, linoleamide MEA, myristamide DEA, oleamide DEA, stearamide MEA, or TEA-lauryl sulfate.

* Styrene acrylates copolymer, which are used as coloring agents in cosmetics and other products. On labels, they're listed as styrene acrylates copolymer, styrene-butadiene copolymer, polystyrene, styrene copolymer, styrene resin, ethylbenzene, or vinylbenzene.
* Lead, antimony, and other heavy metals

FATAL CONVENIENCES: ANTIAGING CREAMS

Here is a perfect example of my problem with modern conveniences. There are tried-and-true ways to slow down how our bodies age. We just need to drink plenty of clean water, eat a healthy, mostly plant-based, whole-food/non-highly-processed diet, get enough physical activity, sleep eight hours a night, and keep up meaningful social connections.

Do all that, and you'll not only look as youthful as possible, you'll feel that way, too. But that sounds like work. It requires effort and commitment for the rest of your life. There must be an easier, more convenient way, right?

Well, there is, but only if you believe the absurd claims found on antiaging potions and lotions. These products prey on our desire for a quick fix, for the magical concoction of chemicals we can purchase in a drugstore and thereby avoid all the sensible, natural paths to maintaining youthfulness.

It's no surprise that we focus most of our antiaging efforts on our skin, the most superficial part of our bodies. If we can knock a decade or two off our faces, we're satisfied and see no need to do anything further.

There's nothing new about our willingness to try just about anything to stop looking our age. Cleopatra supposedly bathed in donkey milk every day because she believed it softened and exfoliated her skin. To do so, she maintained a stable of seven hundred donkeys, which doesn't sound too convenient to me. Women in Elizabethan England put thin slices of meat onto their faces to prevent wrinkles. No thanks!

Today's solutions sound more scientific, but they also expose us to health hazards unknown back in the early days of antiaging wizardry.

The ingredients that make these products hazardous to your skin *and* your health aren't the alleged antiaging components, which are usually either antioxidants or harmless alpha hydroxy acids such as citric acid, hyroxycaprylic acid, or hydroxycapric acid (and sometimes retinol, a form of vitamin A). The FDA tests these products, and aside from making skin more sensitive to UV rays, there seems to be little in them to worry about, except an FDA warning about products from overseas that may be contaminated with mercury. Instead, it's the substances *added* to the mix—stuff that makes the lotions and creams easy to apply and keeps them shelf stable—that create the most potential for harm.

One culprit is the "forever chemicals" PFOAs and PFASs. These, you will remember, are present in thousands of products we use in our daily lives. In antiaging creams, they have been found as contaminants of another class of chemicals, polytetrafluoroethylene (PTFE), present in big brands. They make things smooth and slippery, which sounds useful when you're talking about youthful skin.

But PFOAs have been linked to several cancers (including ovarian and breast), thyroid disease, high cholesterol levels, and disruptions of the endocrine system—none of which sounds worth the promise of softer skin. And we have no way of knowing if our products contain these substances, because contaminants aren't listed among the ingredients.

Okay, So What Should We Do?

The best option, as I started by saying, is to take care of your health by adopting good habits and abandoning bad ones. You can do that now. I have created programs where after three weeks of hydrating, eating right, and exercising, people literally come alive. You can see it everywhere, including in their skin and eyes.

Be grateful for the fact that you're aging. I don't care how many wrinkles you have, it's a lot better than the alternative.

What can we do? Avoid anything containing PTFE, polyperfluoromethylisopropyl ether, or DEA-C8-18 perfluoroalkylethyl phosphate on the label. Frankly, I don't understand how anyone could knowingly put substances with names as long and scary as those on their skin. But I think people make a habit of never reading labels—what you don't know can't hurt you, right? Anyway, it's too much work, and we never understand them (until now!).

According to the Campaign for Safe Cosmetics' Red List, we should stay away from antiaging products or moisturizers containing placental extracts, which can contain progesterone or estrogen; UV filters such as octinoxate, oxybenzone, or homosalate; and petrolatum, for possible polycyclic aromatic hydrocarbon (PAH) contamination.

Anything containing fragrance, parabens, 1,4-dioxane, or polyethylene glycol (PEG) is also risky and should be shunned.

No one actually needs any of these products, for the simple reason that they don't do much aside from making users poorer and preying on those who are insecure about their looks. Do you honestly believe a magic potion capable of defying biology, the aging process, and the passage of time can be found in a plastic tube? It's like Ponce de León believing he could discover the fountain of youth. Instead, all he wound up with was Florida.

Follow these suggestions, and you won't need any product that calls itself "antiaging," even if such a thing existed, which it doesn't. The only guaranteed antiaging product is death: after you die, you'll never be a day older.

FATAL CONVENIENCES: SHAMPOO

We're all a little weird about our hair.

Unlike skin or teeth, it doesn't serve a very important role in our well-being. It protects our scalp from the sun, true, and keeps some body heat from escaping during winter. If the need arises, it provides a little cushioning for our skulls, where our delicate brains reside. Did I leave anything out? But all of us, men as well as women, attach a great deal of importance to the state of our hair. It's a symbol of animal good health and youthful vitality. The thicker and more lustrous it is, the more beautiful and powerful we feel. Good hair is sexy!

We don't only demand that it looks amazing—it ought to smell great, too, and feel silky and soft, if the commercials are to be believed. Bouncy, too? Sure, why not? Anything, as long as it makes us irresistible. So it's no surprise that we spend huge sums on the care and feeding of our follicles, on gels, mousses, sprays, waxes, creams, ointments, and various other products, not to mention bleaches, dyes, tints, and on and on.

We can credit (or blame) our hair lust on the shampoo manufacturer John Breck, who, back in 1929, hired an artist to draw pictures of women with fabulous hair for his ads. Modern formulations were first introduced in the 1930s with Drene, which got rid of oiliness using synthetic chemicals called surfactants instead of plain old soap. In the 1950s, the chemist and salon owner Jheri Redding created the first "crème rinse conditioner," which used protein to repair split ends and other damage caused by, among other things, overwashing.

But not everything in shampoo and conditioner promotes clean, healthy hair. One chemical isn't even listed on the label. It's not an ingredient, technically speaking—it's a by-product of the manufacturing process. Known as 1,4-dioxane, it's been found in more than eighty shampoos, cosmetics, and other products. A 2016 report by the National Institutes of Health's National Toxicology Program says that 1,4-dioxane is "reasonably anticipated to be a human carcinogen based on sufficient evidence of carcinogenicity from studies in experimental animals." The EPA has also classified 1,4-dioxane as "likely to be carcinogenic to humans."

It's impossible to know for certain which shampoo brands contain it, but ingredients associated with it include sodium laureth sulfate, polyethylene glycol (PEG), polyethylene, polyoxyethlene, and all chemicals that end with *oxynol*. Being careful about using shampoo won't necessarily protect you from 1,4-dioxane, however; the EWG has also found it in tap water in forty-five states, serving 90 million Americans.

Another substance to look out for is cocamide DEA, a foaming agent derived from coconut oil, which might lead you to think that it's harmless. But it's not—in 1986 it was added to the state of California's list of substances found in consumer products that might cause cancer, birth defects, or other reproductive harm. The FDA claims there's no reason to worry about it, but it also provides a list of common ingredient names related to this chemical: cocamide DEA, cocamide MEA, DEA-cetyl phosphate, DEA-oleth-3 phosphate, lauramide DEA, linoleamide MEA, myristamide DEA, oleamide DEA, stearamide MEA, TEA-lauryl sulfate, and triethanolamine.

I've even found cocamide in a so-called clean shampoo! Here's a tip: if your shampoo makes a luxuriant amount of suds, beware. Bubbles mean trouble.

Shampoo may also contain other chemicals that are potentially toxic or carcinogenic or act as endocrine disruptors. They include:

+ Preservatives such as parabens, formaldehyde, ketoconazole (an anti-dandruff ingredient and potential endocrine disrupter), and methylisothiazolinone (an allergen that's also toxic to aquatic life)
+ Selenium sulfide, an antidandruff chemical that the National Cancer Institute says is "reasonably anticipated to be a human carcinogen"
+ Fragrance, unless the label identifies which individual chemicals are used

The use of dry powder to clean hair isn't new—in fact, back in Elizabethan days, before running water, people put powder onto their hair to reduce its oil and odor. Today, there is dry shampoo—an alcohol- or starch-based product in a spray can that soaks up the oil rather than washing it away. But if the propellant contains isobutane, it might also be contaminated with the carcinogen benzene. This is why anything using an aerosol spray is best avoided.

Okay, So What Should We Do?

First, recognize that unless you've been rolling around in the mud, your hair probably isn't dirty—and what makes it feel oily isn't oil, it's sebum, the waxy substance our bodies produce to protect our skin. The surfactants in shampoo are what permit the soap to wash the sebum away, but keep in mind that as we age, our follicles dry out, which is why most of us don't need to shampoo more than once a week. Using less shampoo will also spare us some chemical exposures.

Second, accept the fact that shampoo is just soap, not a magic potion. You can use any simple, basic soap on your hair, including the same kind you use on your body, and get good results. Mountains of lather don't mean that your hair is getting any cleaner, shinier, bouncier, or sexier. It could just mean that you're being dosed with chemicals you should avoid. So don't fall for the hair hype.

Though hair thickness and texture are mostly genetic, taking care of your body will also make your hair look healthy. Follicles need protein, minerals, and vitamins, and nutritional deficiencies affect hair growth and quality. UV rays and cigarette smoke can also damage hair. Another way to ensure healthy hair is to maintain proper weight; research from Japan found that obesity can lead to depletion of follicle stem cells, resulting in hair loss.

5

FOOD AND BEVERAGES

ONCE UPON A TIME, WHEN WE wanted to eat, we first had to expend energy, whether by foraging for wild fruits, nuts, roots, and so on or by hunting animals, killing them, and butchering them. In other words, we had to do a lot of work. That fact of life maintained the balance between the calories we consumed and the calories we burned and was one of the reasons there were no obese cavemen or -women or any who suffered from type 2 diabetes, heart disease, or the other food-related ailments. The food was also all natural, unprocessed, organic, and wild, as nature intended.

But it was not at all convenient.

Today, thanks to the invention of agriculture twelve thousand or so years ago, plus the technological advances that have come ever since, you can sit on your sofa and acquire food by burning only the energy required to move your fingers around your phone.

What kind of food is a completely different matter. Agriculture is what makes it possible for the planet to sustain billions of people and enables us all to eat and drink as effortlessly as we do. But the conveniences of easily accessible food have gone overboard. As a result our current food environment, including the healthiest things we can eat, has been transformed, and not always for the better.

When I checked while writing this book, this was the ranking of top sources of calories in the American diet:

1. Grain-based desserts, meaning not only cookies, cakes, doughnuts, and pies but also granola bars, which are essentially desserts in disguise
2. Bread
3. Chicken
4. Soda, energy drinks, and sports drinks
5. Pizza
6. Alcohol
7. Pasta

Notice a pattern there? Nearly everything is made with refined grains, meaning foods that don't require refrigeration and don't spoil. Thanks to modern technology, they don't even get stale the way they once did. A loaf of bread that's as fresh after a month in your kitchen as it was the day you bought it should make you worry.

Invariably, along with those refined grains comes sugar in one form or another; industrialized fats and oils, too. Basically, you're looking at the Standard American Diet, also known as SAD for good reason. Pretty much all that stuff is as convenient as can be, meaning it provides energy consumed with virtually no energy expended, not even the effort required to chop vegetables or turn on a stove.

As we see throughout this book, convenience always comes with a price. Here, it's obesity, diabetes, coronary artery disease, high blood pressure, several types of cancer, liver disease, years of infirmity, and premature death. Astronomical health care costs, too—don't forget that one.

Pass the corn chips, baby!

It's easy to blame individuals for their poor nutritional choices, but we all inhabit the same food environment, over which we have little or no control. And although it's possible to follow a healthy diet, it requires time, knowledge, and effort, all of which are in short supply these days. We (and our kids) are inundated with messages about how great that ultracheesy stuffed crust meat lover's pizza tastes or how great it will be to sink our teeth into a flame-broiled double bacon cheddar burger and then wash it down with a quart of carbonated liquid candy.

But ask somebody what to do with a head of broccoli, a couple cloves of garlic, and a little olive oil, or cranberry beans, tomatoes, and a handful of herbs and spices, and they come up empty. There are kids today who don't recognize some vegetables in the raw because they've never seen them or watched anybody cook them.

As always, the hidden culprit is the profit motive. Modern companies have to grow if they want their stock prices to rise, and how can a food manufacturer stimulate continuous growth? Either by getting us to spend more money on the food we eat (a hard sell) or by getting us to buy more today than we did yesterday and more tomorrow than we did today. That's the mentality that treats food as just another commercial product to be sold to suckers rather than the gift of nature that sustains us and keeps us healthy and thriving.

Which is what food truly is—or should be.

The author Jared Diamond called the switch from hunting and gathering to agriculture "the worst mistake in the history of the human race." Once we shifted away from a diet of natural, whole, unrefined foods—meat, fish, milk, eggs, fruit, vegetables, nuts—to one based on grains, we as a species became shorter and weaker and more vulnerable to inflammation and disease.

I'd call that a fatal convenience, wouldn't you?

FATAL CONVENIENCES: FRUITS AND VEGETABLES

We're not at the point—not yet at least—where we need to fear produce for the hidden hazards and dangerous additives that exist in just about everything else we consume. Apples still contain just one ingredient: apple. The same is true of all the rest of the foods that grow in dirt or hang from trees and bushes. So we feel safe when we eat what we now like to call a "whole-food, plant-based" diet. But that doesn't mean things are as simple and safe as they once were.

Our relationship with fruit and vegetables used to be much more intimate. In 1862, around 90 percent of Americans made their living from the land. That year, President Lincoln signed legislation creating the US Department of Agriculture (USDA), but he also approved the Homestead Act, which eventually put a huge amount of farmland into the hands of agriculture corporations posing as homesteaders.

That was when farming suddenly became a tough business for small operators, and by 1940, only 30 percent of Americans were farmers. Today, the number is 2 percent, despite the fact that the population has boomed and we eat more than ever.

Just as eating has changed—a *lot*—since then, farming has, too, thanks to its own conveniences, mostly technological. In the eighteenth century, it took nearly five acres of land to feed one person for a year. Now that feat is accomplished with just half an acre. You could see this as a good thing: if we are growing more crops with fewer farmers, less land, and less labor, we must be more productive than before. But this efficiency has come at a cost, to both our health and that of the planet.

For instance, to make a farm really efficient, it helps to stick with just a few robust crops—preferably one, in fact. But that takes a toll on the soil. When researchers analyzed data for forty-three crops from 1950 to 1999, they showed declines in six key nutrients—protein, calcium, phosphorus, iron, vitamin C, and vitamin B_2—suggesting a trade-off between yield and nutrient content.

Why are the plants we eat suddenly less good for us? It seems that hearty crops—the kind that produce higher yields—are not so efficient at absorbing nutrients from the soil. This has led to a weird problem that emerged only since industrial farming began: malnourished obese people.

It's no easy task to fill acre upon acre with crops that can resist disease and drought and produce high yields. One way is to use chemical help. After World War II, nitrogen-based fertilizers became an inexpensive solution to increase crop production, and their use has increased dramatically since then. When farmers use nitrogen, it breaks down into nitrate and is absorbed into the groundwater, which can end up in drinking water. Research showed that in agricultural areas, the water in 22 percent of private wells exceeds the safe level of nitrate. Ingesting high levels of nitrate in water increases the rates of thyroid abnormalities in children, studies have shown. In 2006, researchers concluded that nitrate ingested as a result of agricultural runoff is probably carcinogenic.

And just because a fertilizer is all natural doesn't mean it's harmless. Manure isn't carcinogenic, but it *is* a natural home to *E. coli* bacteria, which can cause serious illness and even death. Every year there are recalls of packaged vegetables, usually ones we eat raw, such as lettuce, that have been contaminated with *E. coli*. Though this can happen even on small farms, the problem becomes a lot bigger when produce comes from a gigantic factory farm. *E. coli* from manure has also been found in water used to irrigate crops. In 2018, *E. coli* contamination of romaine lettuce was traced back to an industrial cattle farm. It killed five people and landed ninety-six in the hospital, twenty-seven of whom had kidney failure. Experts say that the cattle waste somehow ended up in the irrigation water.

Then we get to the eight-hundred-pound gorilla in the produce bin: the weed killer, or herbicide, glyphosate, better known by its brand name, Roundup, and the genetically modified organisms that the toxic chemical has brought into existence. Here's where things get really gnarly. Glyphosate has become the most commonly used weed killer in the world since its introduction in 1974. But it works only because certain crops, such as soy, have been genetically modified so that they can resist the chemical's killing power, thereby allowing farmers to spray it at will. But as the weeds have also become resistant, farmers have had to use even more.

Why does this matter? Because glyphosate has been linked to endocrine-disrupting activity, hypertension, diabetes, stroke, autism, kidney failure, Parkinson's disease, and Alzheimer's disease. In 2015, the International Agency for Research on Cancer declared it a probable human carcinogen.

It gets worse: the FDA disagreed with that finding and maintains that glyphosate poses no risk to our health. Here we go again, with the FDA seemingly not looking out for us. Meanwhile, in 2018, a lawsuit against Monsanto, the maker of Roundup, resulted in the public release of documents showing that the company had interfered in the peer review process of academic papers, ghostwritten articles in toxicology journals, and created fake academic websites defending its products.

There's a chance that the tide may be turning. In June 2022, a US Court of Appeals overturned the EPA's decision that glyphosate is safe, forcing the agency to reassess its evaluation. Personally, I don't need to wait for the EPA, the FDA, the USDA, or any other government agency to tell me that I'm better off without glyphosate—or any pesticide, really—in my life.

How About the Environment?

Pesticides and herbicides help farmers grow more robust crops, but these chemicals have also been linked to the death of an important part of our food cycle: bees. They pollinate our crops, so the drastic decline in bee populations over the last few years is extremely concerning. Researchers point to a widely used group of pesticides called neonicotinoids as a possible culprit. Bees are exposed to them in pollen, nectar, dust, and dew on leaves. Neonicotinoids interfere with their nervous system and can lead to paralysis and death. A single treated corn seed contains enough pesticide to kill more than eighty thousand bees. If we blatantly go against nature, there will be consequences. I will continue to hammer at this point: what hurts you will hurt nature, and vice versa.

The use of Roundup to kill weeds isn't just bad for bees; it has also been linked to the sad fate of the monarch butterfly, whose main food source, the milkweed, has been decimated by the herbicide. Without this important source of nourishment, migrating monarchs have been dying off; their population in North America has dropped by as much as 90 percent in the last two decades.

Fertilizer used on industrial farms is also a major contributor to greenhouse gas emissions. Nitrous oxide (N_2O) emissions from farm fertilizers accounted for 74 percent of total N_2O emissions in 2020, and the impact of a pound of N_2O on warming the atmosphere is almost three hundred times that of a pound of carbon dioxide.

Even without those harmful chemicals, modern farming has managed to damage the soil. It's easy to take the health of land for granted—but we forget that it's a living organism, not simply dirt, which is a misnomer in any case.

When early Americans began farming, the soil of the Midwest was thriving. Prairie grass that died and decomposed fed an ecosystem of microorganisms flourishing beneath the top layer of black earth—perfect for growing crops. But after decades of monoculture farming, most of the fertile topsoil in the upper Midwest is gone—depleted. And this has the potential to cause a whole cascade of other problems, as we saw during the Dust Bowl of the 1930s. Scientists estimate that if our current rate of soil loss continues, all of the world's topsoil could be gone in sixty years. That will make eating a healthy, all-natural plant-based diet a thing of the past.

Okay, So What Should We Do?

First things first: we need to continue eating fresh, natural, unprocessed fruit, vegetables, nuts, seeds, mushrooms, and beans. A lot. But we also need to be conscious consumers. Today, we as individuals have many ways to avoid supporting Big Agriculture's bad habits and to improve our health and the environment's, too.

The farmers' market movement has spread to almost every big city, suburb, and small town in the United States. When you shop at one, you support local, small-scale growing, which is usually done using responsible, sustainable methods. You put your money into the pockets of people who live near you. You also cut down on a lot of shipping mileage, because now your berries are coming from thirty or forty minutes away instead of from another continent. You end up buying a lot less plastic, too, since your fruits and vegetables are probably sold naked, without packaging or containers. You're doing the planet a big favor.

But if you *really* want to go local, start an organic garden in your backyard. If you have enough space to get serious about it, that's great. Organizations such as Food Not Lawns (foodnotlawns.com), Green America (greenamerica.org), and Food Forest Abundance (foodforestabundance.com) can help you transform your pretty but pointless lawn into something that produces food for you and your neighborhood insects and other animals. When you realize that US lawns consume roughly 3 trillion gallons of water and 70 million pounds of pesticides a year, you see how much of a difference we can make if we try.

What if we started growing food in some of that? We could solve so many food insecurity issues. Wouldn't it be empowering for you and your family to just walk outside and eat from your yard?

You can feed your family for several months at minimum, more if you get into canning and jarring. If all you can manage is some herbs in a pot or window box or some lettuces in a hydroponic garden, that's great, too, because fresh herbs and greens pack a powerful nutritional punch. You'll have no questions about where your food was grown, how the soil was treated, or whether harmful chemical fertilizers and pesticides were used; your produce won't produce a carbon footprint due to its being shipped or refrigerated in trucks as it travels to you; there won't be containers of any kind, even so-called recyclable ones, to discard; there won't be drives to the supermarket, which take their toll on the air you breathe. And you will be eating food just minutes after it was picked. There's nothing fresher, better tasting, or better for you.

Here's another way I love to make accessible, healthy food: buy organic seeds, such as broccoli, kale, alfalfa, lentils, and so on, and grow sprouts, which are an insanely powerful source of the nutrients those vegetables contain—even more than the mature vegetables. They're cheaper, too. All you need to do is soak the seeds for about eight hours in a jar covered with a square of cheesecloth held in place by a rubber band. Pour out the water, rinse the seeds, refill the jar with water, and stand it upside down at an angle so all the water drains out. Repeat twice a day until the seeds have sprouted. They're amazing in salad. And you just grew yourself a superfood.

Legumes are an important source of plant protein, which is extremely important if you've made the healthy decision to at least decrease the amount of meat and poultry you consume. Buy dried lentils and beans in bulk, then soak and cook them as needed; it's much better than buying them canned, with all kinds of additives, preservatives, and unnecessary chemicals and more containers to throw away.

Remember always to wash produce, even things you peel before eating, such as avocados, cucumbers, and melons. This way you'll be sure to remove as much pesticide residue as possible.

Start paying attention to where your produce was grown. This is part of a larger problem—our insistence on eating fruits and vegetables whether they're in season where we live or not. Once upon a time, you could find certain items only at particular times of year—when they were in season. Today, you can find pretty much anything at any time. But this is possible only because of modern transport, which requires harvesting produce before it's fully matured, so it can reach far-flung shoppers before it's overripe.

The problem with that is twofold: early harvesting means that the nutrients haven't had time to fully develop, so you're being cheated out of antioxidants and so on. And the carbon footprint of produce that travels thousands of miles is killing us. Here's some good advice: eat food only when it's in season where you live! If you have to do without blueberries in February, deal with it. Find something else that you like.

Even better, buy frozen fruits and vegetables. Chances are they were picked at their peak maturity, meaning they're probably even healthier than fresh. Cheaper, too. Don't be a produce snob!

We'd all be a lot safer and healthier if we could eat organic produce only, but there's a problem: it's expensive. Most families couldn't afford all the fruits and vegetables they need if they shopped only organic. But the Environmental Working Group provides a partial solution. It's called the

Dirty Dozen, a list of the produce types that contain the most pesticide residue. If you buy those fruits and vegetables organic and buy conventional produce otherwise, you'll be sparing yourself and your family a lot of possible harm.

The current Dirty Dozen, according to the EWG:

+ Strawberries
+ Spinach
+ Kale
+ Nectarines
+ Apples
+ Grapes
+ Bell and hot peppers
+ Cherries
+ Peaches
+ Pears
+ Celery
+ Tomatoes

On the EWG website (ewg.org), you can find an extended list of what's safe to eat and what's not.

FATAL CONVENIENCES: DAIRY PRODUCTS

I'm a mammal. You are, too, and the main thing we mammals have in common is this: we need milk.

We need it immediately after we're born, for sure, and a little while thereafter. Milk is one of nature's coolest miracles—it contains just the right amount of the proper nutrients (protein, fat, carbohydrates, calcium, vitamins) to sustain a newborn with no other food necessary, and it arrives along with baby free of charge.

But then comes the time when we outgrow our need for milk, roughly when we're able to start eating whole foods. We even stop making lactase, the enzyme that enables us to digest dairy properly. This is nature's way, and if you need proof, ask yourself if you've ever seen any other adult mammal drinking milk.

So how is it that we humans have retained our taste for it? Our agrarian ancestors had good reason to keep drinking milk into adulthood: it is highly nutritious, and historically, if you owned a cow in her reproductive years, it was like having a food factory that required only grass for fuel. But in order to digest dairy products more easily, we began processing milk, turning it into foods such as cheese, butter, yogurt, kefir, lassi, labneh, the list goes on and on—culturing milk to make it edible for all but the most lactose intolerant.

Here in the United States there's another reason we continue to consume milk: we have a whole lot of dairy farmers, which is why the federal government promotes it. If you look at the USDA's MyPlate guide to nutrition, dairy products get their own spot; the official, slightly insane recommendation is that adults consume three cups every day. The USDA oversees something called the National Fluid Milk Processor Promotion Program, which pushes milk as a generic product—you may remember its "Got milk?" ads. Its goal is to foster "a new generation of milk drinkers."

But do we really need more milk drinkers? Is all that dairy—or any dairy at all—good for us?

We're not content to produce milk as nature intended. In 1993, the FDA approved Posilac, Monsanto's synthetic growth hormone, for use in dairy cattle. It contains bovine somatotropin, or bST, which increases cows' milk production, and is given to them a couple months after they've given birth. The FDA says it's safe for both the cows and the humans consuming their milk.

But if that's true, why did both the European Union and Canada ban its use? Their concern is that milk from bST-treated cows has higher levels of something called insulin-like growth factor 1 (IGF-1), a hormone that may increase cancer cell growth. The American Cancer Society says that some early studies found a connection between IGF-1 and the development of prostate, breast, colorectal, and other cancers. In 2019, Spanish researchers conducted a study that covered nearly 850,000 people and found that although there "are some data indicating that higher consumption of dairy products could increase the risk of prostate cancer, the evidence is not consistent."

Well, that's good enough for me! Is there any reason to drink milk that's not outweighed by even the slightest possibility of getting cancer as a result? We all need calcium and the rest of the good things milk contains, but there are safer ways of getting them. Broccoli and broccoli sprouts, beans, nuts, seeds, dark leafy greens, sweet potatoes, and more all contain high levels of calcium.

There's also another issue with bST: its use increases the incidence of mastitis, an infection of breast tissue in dairy cows that's treated with antibiotics. That's bad because overuse of antibiotics in farming and elsewhere creates the possibility of future resistance to the drugs, meaning that someday we'll have a harder time fighting off infections. And the tougher the fight, the stronger the antidote needs to be, creating a cascade of perils.

Finally, I think the whole process of dairy farming is disgusting. Newborn calves are torn away from their mothers, which, as you can imagine, causes both animals distress. According to Austrian researchers, "Cattle are herd animals. As expected, all animals, whether they were reared with or without mothers, produced higher levels of the stress hormone cortisol when being isolated from the herd." All this so we can have milk in our coffee or ice cream for dessert? I just don't get it.

How About the Environment?

As I've mentioned elsewhere, factory farms that house many thousands of large animals in cruel conditions are bad for the environment, the animals (duh), and existence itself. By now we all know this is true, and it's time to stop acting as though we don't. Making it even worse, we waste a huge amount of the milk we do produce. According to the USDA, more than 48 billion pounds of milk were sold in the United States in 2017, with more than 99 million pounds, or 12 million gallons, wasted—spoiled before it could be consumed. At the height of the pandemic, the *New York Times* reported that midwestern farmers were dumping thousands of gallons of unsold fresh milk into lagoons and manure pits. That just makes it all seem even more disgraceful. How dare we do this! We torture these animals to get it, pump them full of chemicals, rip their babies away, and then have the audacity to waste their milk.

Okay, So What Should We Do?

We can learn to live without dairy products. The trend is already going in that direction; consumption of fluid milk is way down from its peak, even though we're eating more cheese and yogurt than ever.

If you still need milk, make sure it's the best, most natural kind. Buying raw, unpasteurized milk is illegal in most places, I believe. But it *is* safe to buy dairy from small, organic producers that raise cows fed on grass only. Make sure your dairy products are clearly marked as being from animals not treated with the hormones rBST or rBGH. And even though use of antibiotics is waning in the milk business, it's still out there. As with all agricultural products, the closer to your home it is produced, the fresher and more sustainable it's probably going to be.

I am not here to tell you what to do, what to consume. I don't judge you at all. What I do want to share with you is the truth so that you can make more informed choices and we all can come together and demand better ways of doing things, better systems, better food, better products, and more humane practices.

Try plant-based milks, which aren't really milk but pack nutritional value all the same. True, only soy has comparable protein. And yes, vitamins A and D must be added, but after milk is pasteurized, it, too, needs the same fortification. So that's a wash. Lots of plant milks also contain sugars, thickeners, emulsifiers, and other unnecessary "improvements," so watch out for those. The best bet in this category is probably organic soy milk.

If you're still living under the illusion that milk is the champion source of calcium, think again. You can get the same amount of that important mineral by eating a cup and a quarter of spinach or black beans as you can from a cup of milk—and without the saturated fat, calories, or cruelty.

FATAL CONVENIENCES: MEAT, POULTRY, AND EGGS

My diet is fully plant based and has been for more than fifteen years. I don't eat any of the things we're about to discuss.

But I can tell you where the dangers lie without saying that you should drop all these foods from your diet completely—even though that's what I believe. I'm not the food police, and I don't want to tell you what to eat or not eat. I just see broken systems and toxic, poor-quality food that's causing problems for people, animals, and the environment.

Obviously, we've been eating animal foods forever, since the first hunter hurled a spear at a fellow wild living thing and brought it home for dinner (and I don't mean as a guest). Meat provided us with necessary nutrients and kept us alive, so it's hard to find fault with that. And we killed only what we needed. Animals eat other animals, too, after all.

At some point along the way, we invented agriculture, which came to include domesticating animals so we could breed them in order to kill and eat them. From then on, things have gone downhill, with factory farming, appalling cruelty, and irresponsible practices that harm the people who eat animals and devastate our environment, thereby hurting everybody else, too, including those of us who never eat meat.

I'm not going to get into the nutritional pros and cons of eating animal foods in this book. You're probably aware of the ongoing dietary warfare among various factions—from my fellow vegans and vegetarians to omnivores to followers of the keto diet all the way down to the hardcore carnivores, who eat practically nothing *but* meat and claim to be in perfect health.

I just want to talk about the Fatal Convenience of meat.

We all know the importance of getting enough protein in our diet to maintain sufficient lean body mass and support all our various physio-logical functions. The easiest way of fulfilling our need for protein, we've been led to believe, is by slapping a big steak onto the grill or sticking a chicken into the oven—or, more probable today, devouring a fast-food burger or some chicken nuggets. That's the convenience part of the equa-tion; there's nothing easier than relying on meat or poultry to supply this necessary nutrient.

Of course, protein isn't all that meat supplies. Eating a steady diet of meat that's been raised by conventional methods—meaning factory farms and all the horribleness that entails—has been credibly linked to heart disease and various cancers, the number one and number two killers of Americans. We eat way more meat than is necessary or healthy, and we suffer big time as a result. Livestock animals aren't the only creatures dying due to our appetite for meat. But not all the dangers are readily apparent.

When vast numbers of animals are crowded into tight spaces, as is common, diseases spread quickly and easily, which is why farmers began administering antibiotics. But they discovered a side benefit of doing so: animals that were given the drugs put on more weight in less time, mean-ing that the farmers made greater profits. Unfortunately, the antibiotics were passed on to humans, and there began to be a surge in antibiotic-resistant superbugs. The FDA acted quickly (for a change) and banned the nonmedical use of penicillin and tetracycline in farm animals. But due to pushback from the farm lobby, the ban has never really been enforced. This is worrisome because antibiotic-resistant bacteria cause more than 2.8 million infections and 162,000 deaths in the United States each year.

Since the 1950s, the FDA has also allowed hormones to be given to cattle and sheep to promote rapid growth. The European Union, however, banned the use of hormones in farm animals back in 1981, fearing that their use could have "endocrine, developmental, immunological, neuro-biological, immunotoxic, genotoxic and carcinogenic effects" on humans, particularly prepubescent children.

The FDA contends that the levels of hormones given to farm animals would be expected to have no harmful effect in humans based on extensive scientific study and review. However, a University of Rochester study examined beef consumption among pregnant women and then measured sperm concentration in their grown sons. They found that men whose moms had eaten the most beef had a sperm concentration that was 24 percent lower than those whose mothers had eaten less, suggesting that the hormones given to cattle might harm testicular development on fetuses in the womb.

Beef, poultry, and eggs, because of the way they're farmed and handled, are all vulnerable to infection by dangerous pathogens such as *E. coli*, salmonella, and other bacteria. You may recall the famous 1986 outbreak of mad cow disease, which attacks the brains of cattle, killing them. You might not realize that when humans eat infected meat, they can come to suffer from Creutzfeldt-Jakob disease (CJD), which is always fatal.

But all those health hazards have nothing to do with meat, poultry, or eggs per se—they're all caused by how Big Meat treats its products and by extension its customers: you.

How About the Environment?

So much has already been said and written about the industrial meat complex's cruelty to living creatures that I can't really think of anything new to add. I guarantee that if you saw how those animals are treated when they're alive and when they are slaughtered, you would be more likely to puke than to chow down. According to one estimate, the average meat-eating adult has consumed 2,400 entire animals, so just imagine all the merciless horrors and killing that have already been done on your behalf, paid for by your grocery dollars. I'll leave it at that.

Instead, let's think about all the cruelty to the environment that comes from animal agriculture. The technical term for industrial or factory farms is concentrated animal feeding operations, or CAFOs. The idea is to take a large number of animals and confine them in as small an area as possible for their entire lives—eating, pooping, laying eggs, producing milk, and growing fat enough to be slaughtered. These animals don't forage for food, eat bugs, or graze on grass. They are given "feed," often government-subsidized cheap corn and other grains.

According to the Natural Resources Defense Council (NRDC), "The average pig farm grew from 945 animals in 1992 to 4,646 in 2004, with the animals often confined to spaces only slightly larger than their bodies." A large, concentrated feeding operation could have "at least 1,000 beef cattle, 700 dairy cows, 2,500 large pigs, or 82,000 egg-laying hens." What kind of impact do you think that might have on the environment?

According to the NRDC, policy makers have long known that big industrial farms are major polluters, which was why the original 1972 Clean Water Act required the EPA to regulate farms just as it does factories. Unsurprisingly, the law hasn't been enforced; NRDC's decade's worth of research found that "the EPA has left health threats largely unmonitored and lacks basic information" about most industrial farms, "including their location, how many animals they have, and how much waste they produce."

According to a study published in the journal *Nature Food*, 57 percent of agriculture-related greenhouse gas emissions come from producing animal-based feed—not food for us but food to grow animals. The researchers calculated that most of the world's cropland is used to sustain livestock, not people. Roughly 500 million tons of manure are produced annually by factory-farmed livestock and poultry—three times the amount we humans create. Before factory farms, manure was part of the sustainable cycle of a farm. It fertilized the soil. But when so many animals produce so much manure in relatively small spaces, it's no longer beneficial to the soil and needs to be removed.

Where does it go? Into pits. Pools, really. In some cases, it is used as compost or fertilizer, turned into fiber, or even used to create energy. Unfortunately, a lot of it ends up in our water. The EPA says that manure is the primary source of nitrogen and phosphorus in our groundwater, which kills fish and plant life. Manure runoff also introduces harmful bacteria and viruses into water. *E. coli* that seeps into water from manure can lead to deadly infections, especially among children and the elderly. In 2021, cow manure–contaminated water in private wells was the number one cause of gastrointestinal illness in Kewaunee County, Wisconsin, causing 230 of 301 cases that year.

Raising animals also requires a lot of precious water; livestock raising accounts for an estimated 43 percent of all water used in the global food system. Also, keep in mind that grazing animals require a lot of pasture land, which is often cleared by destroying forests.

Okay, So What Should We Do?

I can't resist one last opportunity to answer this question honestly. Stop eating animal foods, or at least begin decreasing the amount you and your family consume. Lots of people now follow the "meatless Monday" regimen, giving up meat one day a week. You'll be healthier, you'll be helping the environment, and you'll be giving your karma a break.

Then, learn how to get your protein elsewhere. Abandon the myth that you can't get complete protein from plant sources. According to the Academy of Nutrition and Dietetics, "Protein from a variety of plant foods, eaten during the course of a day, supplies enough of all indispensable (essential) amino acids when caloric requirements are met." It suggests that regularly consuming beans, lentils, and soy products will ensure that you get all the protein you need.

Beans especially are a tasty and cheap way to do this; an analysis by the World Resources Institute found that beans and legumes cost less than 2.5 cents per gram of protein compared to more than 4 cents per gram for beef and that switching from meat or poultry to beans can significantly reduce agricultural resource use and greenhouse gas emissions. It's a win-win.

If you must eat meat, at least make healthy choices. According to a 2022 study, consumption of grass-fed beef "could exert protective effects against a number of diseases ranging from cancer to cardiovascular disease (CVD) as evidenced by the increased functional omega-3 PUFA and decreased undesirable saturated fats." A UK study found that "access to forage, whether fresh or conserved, is a key influencing factor for meat fatty acid profile, and there is increasing evidence that pasture access is particularly beneficial for meat's nutritional quality."

And buy organic meat, meaning from animals that were not given antibiotics or growth hormones.

Buy eggs from pastured chickens. Researchers at Penn State compared the eggs from chickens who foraged on alfalfa, red and white clover, or mixed cool-season grasses to those from hens fed the type of feed used in factory farms. The natural feed birds' eggs had twice as much vitamin E and long-chain omega-3 fats, more than double the total omega-3 fatty acids, and less than half the ratio of omega-6 to omega-3 fatty acids. Their vitamin A content was 38 percent higher. But the pastured hens were smaller than commercial birds and laid fewer eggs—which is probably why farmers prefer to keep their chickens confined indoors.

For more details on the various labels and certifications, see the EWG's Decoding Meat and Dairy Product Labels page at ewg.org.

FATAL CONVENIENCES: FISH AND OTHER SEAFOOD

Seafood has been a staple for populations living close to water ever since the ancient Egyptians went trolling with spears, nets, and rods, and likely long before then, when we fished with our bare hands. As sources of lean protein, healthy fats, and other important nutrients, aquatic animals are better for us than meat or poultry. Big fish eat little fish for a good reason (aside from the fact that their choices are somewhat limited).

Naturally, we love fish so much that we've totally screwed them up as a source of healthy nutrition. We did so mostly by wrecking their habitats, fresh and salt water. Let's run down the list.

We've long known that mercury spewed into the air by burning coal winds up in our water. And the longer a fish lives, the more mercury it accumulates, which is why big predators—tuna, swordfish, sharks—are the most contaminated with this poisonous heavy metal. But a study of trout and bass in fifty lakes in Idaho, Oregon, and Washington found mercury in all samples, with 11 percent exceeding the amount deemed safe by the EPA.

It's especially harmful to children and babies and can even be fatal. According to the CDC, "Mercury can pass from a mother to her baby through the placenta during pregnancy and, in smaller amounts, through breast milk after birth. Exposure to mercury can affect the infant's brain and nervous system development during pregnancy and after birth." The FDA recommends that pregnant and breastfeeding women completely avoid eating shark, king mackerel, tilefish, swordfish, and tuna and eat freshwater fish like pike, walleye, muskellunge, and bass only in moderation.

But all adults can be harmed if they go overboard with fish. You might remember when the actor Jeremy Piven had to bow out of a Broadway play in 2008; he suddenly had trouble remembering his lines, lost his sense of balance, and had extreme fatigue. It turned out he had mercury poisoning—he had been eating sushi twice a day, and fish, he said, was his only source of protein for twenty years.

We also need to worry about the lethal "forever chemicals." One study found that people who ate the most fish also had the highest levels of three different chemicals that have been linked to cancer, thyroid disease, and other serious ailments. Because of PFASs' persistence in the environment, including bodies of water, fish are a carrier of these chemicals, which we then absorb. The study determined that "seven PFAS were detected in at least 30 percent of participants" and found that shellfish consumption was associated with every PFAS except one.

A study in Norway suggested that fish and shellfish are a major dietary source of three "forever chemicals," contributing "38 percent of the estimated dietary intakes of perfluorooctanoic acid (PFOA), 93 percent of perfluoroundecanoic acid (PFUnDA) and 81 percent of perfluorooctane sulfonic acid (PFOS)."

Wow! That study even blew me away.

The pesticide DDT is no longer manufactured in this country. The same is true of polychlorinated biphenyls, or PCBs, widely used industrial chemicals that have been banned here since 1979 and internationally since 2001. These famously toxic chemicals have been linked to cancer, nervous system damage, reproductive disorders, and disruption of the immune system.

But they still persist in our waters. A study of 540 US rivers found PCBs in 93.5 percent of the samples and DDT in 98.7 percent. They were in higher concentrations in fish from urban than nonurban rivers, and although DDT was detected more frequently, it was at lower levels than PCBs, which exceeded human health cancer-screening values in nearly half the samples. The EPA found that the highest concentrations of PCBs in fish was in the Great Lakes. According to the Environmental Defense Fund, the EPA has issued PCB advisories for more than 2 million lake acres and 130,000 river miles since 2003, meaning that people are urged to limit their consumption of fish from those areas.

A Chinese study found that among seafood eaters, fish contributed 57 percent of dietary intake of DDT and mollusks 38 percent, which means that fish not only hold on to DDT but pass it along to us. PCBs tend to be found in bottom feeders such as striped bass, bluefish, eel, and sea trout, as well as predators such as bass, lake trout, and walleye. Farmed salmon that are fed ground-up fish have higher levels than do wild-caught salmon. And PCBs are slow to go—the Environmental Defense Fund estimates that it can take five or more years for them to dissipate from women's bodies, which is of special concern if you're pregnant, since fetuses can be exposed to these chemicals through the placenta.

Generally speaking, wild-caught fish are healthier for us than farmed fish are (we'll discuss this in detail a little farther down). But most fish we eat today is farmed. It's cheaper, it's better for the environment, and it's easier for producers to control—essentially, we have turned water animals into an industrial product, as we did with land animals. But farmed fish aren't without problems, either. According to the National Oceanic and Atmospheric Administration's (NOAA) Fisheries:

> Fish diseases occur naturally in the wild, but their effects often go unnoticed because dead fish quickly become prey. Disease events can occur in fish farms because 1) fish are reared at higher densities than nature, increasing contact between fish; 2) infected fish are not removed as promptly from the farm as they would be by natural predators; 3) farmed fish are more closely and easily observed than wild fish. Thus pathogens that normally exist in low numbers and do not cause disease in the wild may result in disease in farmed fish.

How About the Environment?

Fishing old school with a pole at your local lake doesn't damage anything, especially if you pay attention to regulations that protect aquatic populations. But commercial fishing is a whole other thing—to satisfy our hunger, a huge amount of harm is being done to the planet, especially the seas. We're devastating the populations of the fish we want to keep on eating, so that at some point seafood may be a rare and costly treat. Modern fishing technology is damaging the rest of the environment, too. Here's how Greenpeace summed it up:

> We've already removed at least two-thirds of the large fish in the ocean, and one in three fish populations have collapsed since 1950. Put simply, there are too many boats chasing too few fish.
>
> Overfishing is threatening food security for hundreds of millions of people and destroying ocean ecosystems worldwide.
>
> In fact, the fishing industry can't even sell everything it catches. One commercial fishing boat, which can be the size of a cruise ship, can catch more fish in one haul than hundreds of small-scale boats can in a year.
>
> Not only is the amount of fish we're catching unsustainable,

the way we're catching it also has serious consequences. As fishing techniques have evolved to catch the most fish possible, they've also become more destructive.

For example, bottom trawling—in which giant nets are run along the sea floor picking up or crushing whatever is in their path—is particularly damaging to fragile coral and sponge habitats. Longlining—a technique that consists of baiting thousands of hooks along miles-long fishing lines—snags thousands of creatures that are typically thrown back into the water dead or dying.

These "unwanted" species, called bycatch, often include turtles, albatross, sharks, manta rays, and even dolphins, many of which are endangered. Every year, commercial fishing kills as many as 300,000 whales, dolphins, and porpoises and about 100 million sharks.

Yes, you read that correctly. This system is so unbelievably broken, it blows me away.

One way to reduce overfishing might be to eliminate government subsidies to the fishing industry. A 2009 study published in the *North American Journal of Fisheries* found that $713 million per year of direct subsidies, or financial support, goes to the US fishing industry, roughly half of which could contribute to overfishing.

"Seas are a critical source of protein for billions of people," the environmentalist Paul Hawken observed. "Small-scale fishing provides work or subsistence harvests to over 100 million people. Over the past three decades, however, the number of overharvested fish stocks have more than tripled due to industrial-scale fishing, risking permanent loss of iconic species such as Atlantic cod, bluefin tuna, and a wide range of sharks. The unchecked expansion of the global fishing fleet, often with government support, is largely responsible for this state of affairs, including destructive harvesting practices like bottom-trawling and shark finning."

Peter Neill, the director of the World Ocean Observatory, wrote, "If we were to declare a moratorium on industrial scale fisheries for a term of five years, we would maintain most of today's fishing-related employment, produce most of the catch that today reaches market for human consumption, reduce fuel costs dramatically, reduce subsidies even more dramatically, and otherwise invest in the future of the industry through its return to health, diversity, and sustainable future supply."

The practice known as bottom trawling—fishing with heavy nets that drag across the seabed—emits roughly the same amount of carbon dioxide as aviation does. The greenhouse gas release isn't just from the boats, it's also because carbon in the seabed is released when the ocean floor is churned up. Even discarded nets are a problem. One study found that 86 percent of the 42,000 tons of plastic in the Great Pacific Garbage Patch was fishing nets.

Okay, So What Should We Do?

According to the Environmental Working Group, our best bets for fish containing healthy omega-3 fatty acids and low levels of mercury are wild-caught salmon, sardines, mussels, rainbow trout, and Atlantic mackerel. These are likely caught using sustainable practices. Also recommended are oysters, anchovies, pollock/imitation crab, and herring. If you catch your own, pay attention to advisories in your area by checking the EPA's fish advisory online database at epa.gov. The agency monitors pollutants and provides recommendations for which fish to avoid or limit.

To reduce exposure to PCBs, don't overdo your consumption of salmon and bluefish, and don't deep-fry fish, because that seals chemical pollutants into its fat. If you eat canned tuna, skip the white and stick with light. *Consumer Reports* tested and found that white albacore tuna contains significantly more mercury than light tuna (but every sample contained mercury). And although the Environmental Defense Fund recommends consuming canned light tuna only and even that less than once a week, *Consumer Reports* suggests that pregnant women avoid it entirely. As an alternative, it recommends canned Alaskan salmon, which is lower in mercury and PCBs.

Keep this in mind when you're thinking of having sashimi or sushi for dinner: according to the Harvard T. H. Chan School of Public Health, "Cooking is known to reduce mercury content in fish by up to 30 percent."

Everybody knows that salmon is extremely healthy, which accounts for its popularity, but then the question is: wild caught or farmed? Consider this:

+ Wild has fewer calories and saturated fat, although farmed has higher levels of omega-3 fatty acids. Winner: wild.
+ PCB levels are sixteen times as high in farmed fish as in wild. Winner: wild.
+ A study from Norway found that farmed salmon had some of the lowest levels of PFASs among 246 fish sampled, while Finnish research claims that wild salmon is one of the highest sources of PFASs in the national diet. Winner: farmed.
+ Mercury levels in salmon are low, and there's not much difference when it comes to wild versus farmed. Winner: tie.

So wild caught looks like the smart choice, but in 2015, the *New York Times* reported that a study using DNA analysis on eighty-two wild salmon samples sold by restaurants and stores found that two-thirds had been mislabeled. The group that conducted the analysis, Oceana, claims that seafood fraud is a big problem in the United States, and encourages citizens to petition the FDA to trace seafood from boat to plate to ensure that it is safe, legally caught, and honestly labeled.

You can also play it safe by eating aquatic flora rather than fauna. Seaweed is a nutritional powerhouse, and the farms actually benefit the ecosystem: they reduce ocean acidification, capture carbon, reduce nitrogen levels and toxic algae blooms, and enhance biodiversity.

Some online resources:

+ NOAA's FishWatch (fishwatch.gov) lets you look up fish to see how depleted each species is, what fishing rules are in place, and the impact fishing has on their habitats.
+ You can also use EWG's Seafood Calculator (ewg.org/consumer -guides/ewgs-consumer-guide-seafood) to get a list of recommendations based on your age and weight.

FATAL CONVENIENCES: PROCESSED FOODS

By now we've been messing around with our food for thousands of years. For most of that time it's been a healthy thing to do.

We fermented, we cultured, we pickled and brined, we salted and dried—we took actions to preserve foods long before we had refrigerators and freezers, so the practice has always had positive goals. Beans and grains would be inedible if we didn't process them first, and without processing we couldn't enjoy hummus, cheese, yogurt, coffee, chocolate, wine, beer . . . the list goes on and on.

So how did "processed food" wind up meaning unhealthy junk?

It's a predictable story. As long as we were processing foods in traditional, old-school ways—meaning as little as possible and always with respect for what we would wind up eating—we were safe. In fact, fermented vegetables like sauerkraut and kimchi are actually more nutritious because of processing.

But then at some point in the twentieth century, the food engineers went to work. They began not just processing foods but inventing totally new edible substances—I call them that because they don't deserve to be called food. The scientists took things found in nature, such as grains and fats, stripped them of everything healthy, added artificial flavoring, dyes, preservatives, and other weirdness, sold them cheaply, and somehow convinced people to eat them.

They are sold in food stores, but they're not food! Doesn't seem to matter to a lot of people.

Enormous marketing budgets capable of blanketing TV time, especially when kids are watching, definitely helped. Making those junk foods what the experts call "hyperpalatable"—meaning better tasting than anything Mother Nature can manage—did the rest. Why eat an ear of fresh organic corn when you can have some unnaturally flavored, ultrasweet/ultrasalty, addictive popcorn instead?

That's how processing food went from being a cool thing to a nutritional nightmare.

Want to know if the purchase you're considering is the evil kind of processed? Easy. Does it have a long list of ingredients, most of which sound as though they belong in a chemistry lab? Is it contained in a brightly colored, beautifully designed bag or box? Is it loaded with sugars or salts and pretty much devoid of fiber, vitamins, and minerals? Are your kids begging you to buy it? Does it have its own TikTok account?

Like I said, it's easy to figure out exactly what we need to avoid. It's common sense. Here are a few of the main culprits that make processed foods so toxic.

Cured meats taste good—but a major part of the curing process is the addition of sodium nitrite or nitrate, which slows down spoilage, improves the flavor, and fends off botulism. Their pink hue is a result of the chemical reaction between the sodium nitrite and the meat proteins. Nitrates are found naturally in fruit and vegetables, but when consumed in cold cuts, they cause problems.

Consumption of processed meat has been linked to an increase in certain types of cancer, including colorectal and stomach, so much so that the American Institute for Cancer Research recommends avoiding them altogether. It found that for every 50 grams (about one hot dog or two slices of ham) eaten daily, the risk of developing colorectal cancer rises by 16 percent. Cured meats have also been linked to hypertension; diabetes;

heart disease; chronic obstructive pulmonary disease, especially among smokers; and higher all-cause mortality.

High-fructose corn syrup (HFCS) can be found in everything from soda to bread. It's essentially ultraprocessed corn designed for powerful sweetness, which makes it a very cheap way to add sugar to just about anything. As HFCS in foods became more common, scientists noticed an increase in obesity, which led to questions of whether humans digest this sweetener differently than we do natural sugar. Between 1970 and 1990, consumption of HFCS increased by 1,000 percent. Eating too much isolated sugar, no matter the source, will increase risk of obesity, cancer, and metabolic diseases.

Margarine, shortening, and palm oil will soften and spoil over time, which was why manufacturers began processing them with hydrogen. Hydrogenation keeps ingredients stable, but it also creates trans fatty acids, or trans fats, which have been shown to increase the risk of heart attacks, stroke, and inflammation. In 2015, the FDA determined that partially hydrogenated oils should be removed from all foods, and now they're no longer used. Fully hydrogenated oils are not as bad as trans fats, but they still contain a lot of saturated fat, which is unhealthy when consumed in large quantities. You can identify them by reading the product label—for instance, it might say either "palm oil" or "hydrogenated palm oil."

Butylated hydroxyanisole (BHA) and butylated hydroxytoluene (BHT) are used as preservatives in some foods because they stabilize fats and prevent them from going rancid. They're also found in breakfast cereals, some desserts, chewing gum, and glazed fruits. According to the National Toxicology Program, BHA is "reasonably anticipated to be a human carcinogen" based on animal studies, though human studies have been inconclusive. But the FDA claims that it's generally recognized as safe for use in food.

Whenever there are conflicting opinions like this, the wise decision is to avoid them. Why take unnecessary chances with your health?

Interestingly, no link has been found between BHT and cancer, and it may actually provide some benefits; a study at New York Medical College found that it might even help prevent the disease.

Titanium dioxide, a powdery white mineral, is in everything from paint to sunscreen to candy, gum, sauces, and pastry; it makes things bright white and prevents spoilage. In 2021, the European Food Safety Authority declared that it's no longer considered safe in food, saying that particles "can accumulate in the body." The worry is that titanium dioxide can damage our DNA and lead to cancer.

When you fry or cook potatoes and certain other foods at high temps, a substance called acrylamide forms through a chemical reaction between the sugars and amino acids. An analysis of thirty-two studies found that among nonsmokers, dietary acrylamide consumption was associated with an increase in endometrial and ovarian cancers. It's what makes potato chips and French fries taste so damn good, but again—is it worth the danger?

Synthetic food dyes, from FD&C Yellow No. 5 to FD&C Red No. 40, are used to create the vibrant colors of everything from candy to cereal to ice cream. The Center for Science in the Public Interest has long petitioned the FDA to ban these dyes because they can increase behavior problems in children, including hyperactivity. Some dyes, including Red No. 3, might also be carcinogenic, while Yellow No. 5 can cause allergic reactions. Europe requires a warning label on foods containing certain dyes, but the FDA hasn't taken similar action here.

Anything that comes in plastic bags or containers that are meant to be heated in the microwave might leach endocrine-disrupting chemicals into your food. A study from 2011 found that plastic containers, even if they're BPA free, still released harmful chemicals. And it's not limited to microwaves—anytime you heat food in plastic you might be releasing estrogenic chemicals. And if you ever microwave butter-flavored popcorn, don't inhale the steam when you open the bag: a study of factory workers showed that the butter-flavored chemical diacetyl, when mixed with air, can cause lung disease. Some food manufacturers have switched from diacetyl to the supposedly safer 2,3-pentanedione, but recent studies have found that it might be just as bad.

How About the Environment?

The problems begin even before we start eating. Those "forever chemicals" I keep bringing up? A study by *Consumer Reports* of more than a hundred food-packaging products found PFASs in everything from paper bags for fast-food French fries and hamburger wrappers to disposable salad bowls and single-use paper plates. It's there so the wrapper doesn't stick to the hot food.

Even packaging that claimed to be moving away from these toxic chemicals still had detectable levels. When PFASs are phased out, it often means that manufacturers are using different chemicals, with no guarantee that they won't do similar damage to us and the environment. According to *Chemical & Engineering News*, "Citing competition, most paper and packaging companies won't discuss the products they're making."

Gee, I wonder why!

In 2022, the FDA banned another harmful ingredient found in fast-food packaging: phthalates, those notorious hormone disrupters. In fact, it banned twenty-three of them. But nine more of the chemicals are still allowed. It never ends.

No matter which evil substances your food packaging contains, it accounts for almost 23 percent of landfill materials. Nearly a quarter! Just look around wherever people gather outdoors, like at beaches, lakes, and parks, and see all the food-related trash—a lot of which winds up in the bellies of the poor birds, beasts, and fish that mistake it for food.

A final environmental hazard associated with processed foods, one that's been getting some attention lately, is the devastation caused by harvesting palm oil. All over the world, forests are being razed and animal habitats destroyed due to the demand for this fat, which is used not only in food but in a long list of personal care products, such as moisturizer. I wish I could offer some advice on how to combat this terrible situation, but the only thing to do is avoid any product containing palm oil.

Okay, So What Should We Do?

As I like to say, it's better to pay the grocer than the doctor and smarter to trust the farmer than the pharmacist.

What I mean is that even though it's slightly more expensive to eat natural food that's only minimally processed (if at all), instead of things that have been mass produced by mammoth industrial corporations, it's worth it in the long run. In the short run, too—you'll feel better and look more beautiful.

A study done in 2013 found that the healthiest diets cost about $1.50 more per day than the least healthy. Even if inflation has made that gap larger, you and your family are worth a couple extra bucks a day.

Speaking of dollars, a big reason our food environment sucks is because most government agricultural subsidies go to corn, soybeans, wheat, and rice—all of which are refined and turned into food that's empty of nutrition and full of chemicals and other junk. If we all contacted our elected officials and complained, maybe federal food policy would become sane. A study found that if the government were to create a subsidy to reduce the price of fruits and vegetables by 10 percent, it would prevent or postpone cardiovascular disease mortality by 150,500 lives by 2030.

But the government isn't going to do its part, so we all have to do ours. When you're shopping at the supermarket, stick to the perimeter, where whole foods such as fruits and vegetables, fish, meat, and dairy products are sold. Don't neglect the frozen food section, where you can find vegetables and fruits picked at their maximum ripeness. This aisle is the frugal shopper's best friend.

In the center aisles, stick with foods that have as few ingredients as possible, and read the labels before you buy. Manufacturers are legally required to tell you all the nasty, unnecessary, toxic junk that's in the "food" they're trying to sell you. Here's a good rule of thumb: if there's an ingredient listed on the label that you couldn't buy on its own, it's probably bad for you.

Remember, just because you can find it in a grocery store doesn't mean you should eat it!

Whenever possible, buy your food close to the source—at farmers' markets and roadside farm stands, for instance. All over the country, small farms are popping up, usually run by idealists who want to grow nutritious produce using natural, sustainable, responsible methods. You may pay a little more, but it's worth it.

My best advice for those who are ready to commit to healthy, budget-friendly eating? Grow your own! Even with a little space you can create an organic garden and enjoy the freshest, cleanest vegetables possible at the lowest cost. If all you have is space for a window box or hydroponic garden, plant some herbs or lettuces.

Now learn to cook all that good food you've grown. When we prepare our own meals, we know exactly what we're eating. And we can take pride in all the wonderful, delicious, healthy things our labors have produced. The more time people spend making food at home, the higher the quality of their diets, common sense tells us and the research proves.

FATAL CONVENIENCES: WATER AND OTHER DRINKS

Our bodies are around two-thirds water, a fact that amazes me every time I think of it. How can water take so many different forms—hair, skin, blood, organs? Even our bones are 30 percent water! We're like walking oceans.

Of course, we all take great care to drink only clean, uncontaminated water to replenish what our bodies lose in the course of a day. Naturally, that attitude extends to the other beverages we consume because, after all, they're mostly water, too.

If only that were true!

Instead, it's now nearly impossible to drink nontoxic beverages. It's not enough to avoid the junk that is obviously bad for our health, such as soda. According to the federal government, most US tap water is contaminated with chemicals proven to cause kidney and testicular cancer, thyroid disease, high cholesterol levels, liver damage, and immune system dysfunction. If we can't trust plain water, we're really in trouble.

How did it come to this? It's because of all the poisons and other junk we release into our environment. Most of the planet is covered in water—so where else could all that garbage we create go except into the drink? All the industrial pollutants, all the exhaust from all the internal combustion engines, every little bit of toxic waste we create—it has to settle somewhere. It settles first in our water, then in us.

According to the CDC, virtually every person ever tested has some PFASs or PFOSs—the "forever chemicals" I keep talking about—in his or her blood. How did they get there? From drinking tap water, most likely. These chemicals have been found in the water supply of more than 2,800 communities in all fifty states, meaning that every day more than 200 million Americans are drinking potentially dangerous toxins—substances that can cause several cancers and a long list of other ailments.

How bad is the situation? In 2022, researchers at the University of Stockholm announced that "based on the latest U.S. guidelines for PFOA in drinking water, rainwater everywhere would be judged unsafe to drink." As I write this, various federal and local agencies say they're going to crack down on the permissible presence of these chemicals in our drinking water. They've been saying that for a while now, but they're not doing much to protect us.

If you thought you were safe because you don't rely on tap water, think again: even well water has been tested and found to be contaminated with these and other shady chemicals. They're everywhere. The EPA compiles a list of tainted sources, including those in private drinking water wells. And a report from the US Geological Survey found industrial toxins in untreated well water in Delaware.

You may have heard about the microbits of plastic that pervade our oceans. But they are also in fresh water, such as rivers. A 2022 study from Northwestern University found microplastic levels in water capable of resulting in ninety thousand pieces of plastic ingested annually by humans from bottled water and four thousand more from tap water, according to calculations. Microplastic consumption can lead to thyroid hormone disruption and may make us obese by altering the way we store fat and burn energy.

Seriously, are we trying to hurt ourselves? The things we expect to be safe, like turning on the faucet, are messing with our hormones!

It's tempting to believe that if we discover an unspoiled natural spring far from civilization, we can drink freely and without fear of contaminants. No way. You should not sip from a natural water source, no matter how perfect it looks. In nature, water travels far, absorbing bacteria, parasites, and viruses along the way. Bottled spring water has been tested and/or filtered in some way to ensure that it's pathogen free.

Lead in water is still a problem, believe it or not, commonly found in the pipes of older homes (which was what happened in Flint, Michigan). Drinking and absorbing too much of this metal can damage kidneys, increase the risk of developing hypertension, and cause reproductive problems. It's also responsible for learning difficulties, lower IQ, and slow growth in children. Even if you live in a newer home with PVC pipes, your child could be drinking water from lead pipes still in use in schools and other old buildings.

Once we go beyond water, the dangers multiply. Now we're dealing with water plus. Soft drinks are a health hazard not only because they're everywhere—is there any place left in America where you can't buy a soda?—but also because they keep growing bigger. Before 1950, the average soft drink was six and a half ounces; today it's twenty. Next time you're at a convenience store, check out the cups at the soda station. They're the size of buckets!

The biggest worry, beyond the artificial colorings and flavorings, is sugar and high-fructose corn syrup. But don't think that "diet" versions get you off the hook. Artificial sweeteners such as aspartame (in Diet Coke) and acesulfame-K (in Diet Pepsi) have both been linked to an increased risk of cancer. Your soda will also probably contain citric acid, added as a preservative and flavor enhancer. All that acidity can damage tooth enamel. For all the calories we try to avoid, the obesity problem isn't getting any better.

Young people especially love sports drinks and energy drinks—anything that comes with the halo of athleticism and good health. Of course, the actual benefits are nonexistent, but the damage they may be doing is real. The original formula Gatorade (not all the variations), a legit electrolyte drink developed by scientists for the University of Florida Gators teams, is just water, sugar, salt, citric acid, and potassium—which is fine if you're doing two-a-day workouts under a broiling tropical sun. It's totally unnecessary otherwise. And it contains Red No. 40 dye. There is virtually no evidence that it hydrates you more than clean water with a pinch of unrefined Himalayan salt. Skip the fake-colored drinks in plastic and just drink the right water.

I've seen estimates that sports drinks make up about 26 percent of youths' sugar-sweetened beverage intake, thereby increasing the risk of obesity, health problems such as type 2 diabetes, and cardiovascular disease. Even gout! Like soda, they can hurt our teeth by increasing the risk of cavities. For most of us, water is good enough for rehydration, unless we're engaging in vigorous exercise for more than an hour and sweating profusely.

Energy drinks often contain large amounts of caffeine; an eight-ounce cup of coffee contains about 100 grams, compared to a can of Monster, a popular brand, which provides 160 grams. The amount of caffeine contained in a cup and a half of coffee is a lot for a kid and can even cause intoxication. Of all caffeine overdoses reported in 2007, nearly half occurred in children under nineteen. There's even some concern that energy drink consumption can increase arterial stiffness in healthy young people, possibly because of the way it raises blood pressure. If you really need to boost your energy artificially, have a cup of coffee.

Of course, we used to think that coffee drinking was an unhealthy habit due to the caffeine. Now that view has changed. Moderate consumption, no more than two or three cups a day, may even be good for us; there's research that links it to lower rates of heart disease, heart failure, arrhythmia, and stroke. It might even protect against neurodegenerative diseases, improve asthma, and lower the risk of certain gastrointestinal diseases. Coffee actually contains antioxidants!

The problem is that nowadays, many of us prefer what are known as "coffee drinks"—a little coffee plus a whole lot of other stuff thrown in, including sugar and flavorings. Of course, we have no idea what's in those flavorings. And the caloric punch these elaborate, expensive drinks pack is huge: a Starbucks Pumpkin Spice Latte, for example, contains 50 grams of sugar, 14 grams of fat, and 380 calories. As a comparison, a sixteen-ounce black coffee contains 5 calories.

I do not drink coffee, and I believe it can be extremely acidic for the body. I get my antioxidants from many other sources, such as fresh green juices, blueberries, cacao, medicinal mushrooms, and others.

How About the Environment?

The global popularity of bottled water created an entirely new level of environmental disaster. According to a 2019 report from the Reuters news agency, every year 481.6 billion plastic water bottles are sold globally—about a million bottles a minute. Fewer than half of the discarded bottles are collected for recycling, and just 7 percent of those are actually turned into new bottles. Most end up in landfills or the ocean. Younger readers might have a hard time believing this, but not so long ago bottled water wasn't even a thing. Somehow we all survived. The problem isn't limited to the bottles; according to a Greenpeace study of 367 waste treatment facilities, their shrink-sleeved labels make most beverage bottles nonrecyclable, so pretty much anything that isn't category PET 1 or HDPE 2 heads to a landfill. Just because you put something into your recycling bin doesn't mean it won't wind up on a huge, nonbiodegradable heap somewhere.

Okay, So What Should We Do?

Drink as much clean water as possible! How's that for a simple solution? Remember, you're mostly water, so you need to replenish what you're constantly losing through breathing, sweating, and urinating. If you feel the need to drink any other beverages, be cautious, because most of the choices available are unhealthy.

As we've seen, we can't trust any of our sources—tap water, well water, bottled water—to be uncontaminated either by bacteria, carcinogens, or other junk. Bottom line: We all need some kind of water filtration setup. Trust me, it's no longer optional. In my home I have a reverse osmosis system, which pumps the water through a series of filters that removes virtually all particles, even the ones too small to see, so all that's left is pure water. I add a pinch of pink Himalayan salt to every glass—I don't taste it, but it remineralizes the water, which is extremely important.

Instead of buying bottled water, get a good nonplastic—glass-lined or metal—bottle and use it. A lot. You'll be doing yourself and the rest of the planet a huge favor. But don't give up on your right to nonpoisonous tap water—we can all agitate for change. On its website, the EPA makes available local Consumer Confidence Reports (epa.gov/ccr), where every municipality must publish an annual water quality report, listing exactly what's in its drinking water, from bacteria to lead to the chemicals used to treat the water. Support legislation and the legislators who are trying to make our water safe again. Reach out to office seekers who are willing to hold industry responsible for polluting our waterways.

When it comes to our health habits, we're so fixated on what we eat that we sometimes forget to think about what we drink. But it all goes into the same body and is of equal importance. A toxin is a toxin, and an unhealthy ingredient is an unhealthy ingredient no matter how you consume it.

According to the CDC, sweetened drinks are the leading source of added sugars in the American diet. Keep that in mind next time you wonder why you can't control your weight. Don't be conned by "sports" or "energy" drinks that use a halo of athleticism to hide the fact that they're full of sugar, caffeine, and other junk no athlete needs. Read labels, and ask yourself if any beverage is going to make you healthier than plain old water. I'm guessing that the answer is no.

6

ELECTROMAGNETIC RADIATION

I'M ABOUT TO PROVE TO YOU that your use of electronic devices—everything from your cell phone to your computer to your Wi-Fi modem and router and Bluetooth and Alexa and every wearable and so-called smart appliance you own—could be causing you physical harm that might result in serious illness and possibly even death.

Okay, that's not exactly true. (Though I can't say for sure it's completely false, either.) Here's my point: If it *were* true, what would you do? Would you throw away all your electronic toys and tools and never touch one ever again? Especially since now you know that failing to do so would put you and your loved ones in terrible danger? Could you live without all that stuff? Would you even try?

Once upon a time, twenty or thirty years ago, the trappings of the digital world were mere conveniences. They were brand-new, totally cool playthings. Today, I can safely say, while typing on a laptop connected to the internet, with my cell phone by my side, that they have become necessities. If we were all to check out of the connected world tomorrow, the global disruption would be catastrophic. It would be as if the planet had suddenly been hurtled back to the Stone Age, or at least to the twentieth century. How would we communicate? How could we share information? Where would we post cat videos?

Compared to the other chapters, this is going to be a weird one.

Throughout this book, I've been sounding the alarm on all kinds of dangers in the products we use every day. This chapter's no different, but the dangers are.

For one thing, they're invisible. For another, they're all around us whether we use them or not. And unlike the chemicals and other substances we've been discussing, when it comes to these Fatal Conveniences, we have no clear idea of which hazards we face, how serious they are, or what—if anything—we can do to make ourselves safer.

We are living in an experiment.

How does that make you feel? It scares me a lot. There's plenty of reason to believe that simply being in the wireless, digital world exposes us to danger. For this, scientific proof definitely does exist. I'm talking about things such as increased risk of leukemia, brain tumors, cancer, and disruption of our reproductive systems. You might not be aware of all the research, but there are reasons for that. We haven't produced nearly enough studies and scientific papers. There are reasons for that, too.

Once you look beyond what little information we do have, the picture gets murky. Technology is advancing so fast that studies done today are outdated tomorrow. Uncovering the influence of invisible radiation and waves is a lot more challenging than determining the effects of chemicals on our bodies. It's to nobody's advantage (except yours and mine) to spend a fortune on credible top-shelf research into this subject.

The government isn't worried about how our health is affected by digital technology. That's why the Federal Communications Commission (FCC) regulates all this stuff rather than the EPA, the CDC, or the FDA. So we've been lulled into a false sense of security. Then there's the simple truth that if our electronics really *are* dangerous, we'd rather not know. Because then we'd have to take some actions that we truly do not want to take.

Once I began working on this chapter, I realized it could easily be a book all on its own. Still, I'm going to try to tell you some things I think you should know.

The first thing to know is that we ourselves run on electricity. Our hearts operate on electrical impulses, and when something goes wrong with the beating mechanism, doctors implant a battery-operated device into our chest to fix the problem. Electrolytes are the minerals such as sodium, potassium, and others containing electrical charges that regulate our cellular activity and keep us alive. Our brains run on electricity.

Long before Ben Franklin flew his kite, or Thomas Edison screwed in a light bulb, or Elon Musk made electric cars cool, electricity played a major role in human existence. We contain it.

But once it began to exist outside our bodies, our relationship started to change. Today, our lives have been completely transformed by electrical conveniences. They gave us light, gave us heat, allowed us to use the hours after dark as we please: to work, to play, to live. We disconnected ourselves from the rhythms imposed by sunlight and seasons, but it felt good.

As conveniences go, electricity and everything it has made possible have been amazing. Nobody sane would want to go without.

But along the way, we created an invisible electrical storm that surrounds us twenty-four hours a day. It's inescapable. It messes up our innate circadian rhythms and affects everything from our sleep patterns to our immune systems to our cellular repair processes.

Part of what makes this topic so hard to understand is all the technical jargon, so let's take care of that now. Start with electromagnetic radiation, or EMR. All your wireless devices create EMR. So does your microwave oven. So does your TV. So does the wiring in your home. EMF is short for electromagnetic field, which means the EMR that surrounds us and has done so since time began. Planet Earth itself creates an EMF. It's why the needle on a compass points north. Everything from electrical power generator lines to your hair dryer creates fields of electromagnetic energy.

There are two basic types of EMR: ionizing and nonionizing. The ionizing kind is powerful, strong enough to bust open atoms and send electrons flying. What makes this kind dangerous is its ability to penetrate deep into human bodies and alter our DNA and our cells. X-rays work because they're ionizing, but that's also why you wear a lead apron in the dentist's chair and why you have to be careful about getting too many body scans. Nuclear explosions are ionizing, too.

The devices we use in our daily lives do not emit this kind of radiation—only the nonionizing, supposedly harmless kind. Most scientists say confidently that nonionizing radiation is safe because it's too weak to penetrate deeply into our bodies and directly damage our DNA or our cells. We have to assume that they're right.

So what's my problem? It's that nobody has proven that over time, nonionizing radiation doesn't *indirectly* damage our DNA and our cells and possibly cause some of the serious, even fatal conditions that I mentioned a few paragraphs ago.

In fact, there's a whole lot of evidence suggesting that electromagnetic radiation might indeed be dangerous in indirect ways that we don't yet understand.

The abstract of a paper published in 2017 in the journal *Environmental Pollution* by a prominent scientist named Magda Havas sums it up nicely:

This paper attempts to resolve the debate about whether nonionizing radiation (NIR) can cause cancer—a debate that has been ongoing for decades. The rationale, put forward mostly by physicists and accepted by many health agencies, is that, *"since NIR does not have enough energy to dislodge electrons, it is unable to cause cancer."* This argument is based on a flawed assumption and uses the model of ionizing radiation (IR) to explain NIR, which is inappropriate. Evidence of free-radical damage has been repeatedly documented among humans, animals, plants and microorganisms for both extremely low frequency (ELF) electromagnetic fields (EMF) and for radio frequency (RF) radiation, neither of which is ionizing. While IR directly damages DNA, NIR interferes with the oxidative repair mechanisms resulting in oxidative stress, damage to cellular components including DNA, and damage to cellular processes leading to cancer. Furthermore, free-radical damage explains the increased cancer risks associated with mobile phone use, occupational exposure to NIR (ELF EMF and RFR), and residential exposure to power lines and RF transmitters including mobile phones, cell phone base stations, broadcast antennas, and radar installations.

Her paper cites a long list of studies that provide scientific reasons to keep asking the question that nags at me: Are we *really* sure that we're not being harmed by the indirect effects of nonionizing radiation?

And the answer is no. We're not *really* sure. We just act like we are. Here's what the World Health Organization has to say on the subject:

Electromagnetic fields (EMF) occur in nature and have always been present on earth. However, during the 20th century, environmental exposure to man-made sources of EMF steadily increased due to electricity demand, ever-advancing wireless technologies and changes in work practices and social behaviour. Everyone is exposed to a complex mix of electric and magnetic fields at many different frequencies, at home and at work, and concern continues to grow over possible health effects from overexposure.

So even a mainstream outfit like the World Health Organization acknowledges that "concern continues to grow over possible health effects from overexposure."

Here's what I think: "overexposure" means that we're getting more than is good for us. But as always happens when human health is up against business interests, human health comes in second. Every page of this book proves that. We're never going to force the tech giants to fund research to find out for sure whether exposure to their products is harming us. Instead, we're all going to have to live with it for years, decades, the rest of our lives, and then—maybe—we'll find out whether it damaged our DNA or our reproductive system, if it caused our cancer, infertility, and other serious malfunctions.

That's how the world works today. It makes no sense to me, either. Technology advances in leaps and bounds, faster than any health researchers can possibly move, which is partly why the science will never catch up. It's like trying to hit a moving target. Tech companies want to innovate and disrupt, to make life easier, faster, and more frictionless than before. That's how billion-dollar fortunes are born. We can't trust those tech bros to carefully evaluate their innovations before they ship them out into the world.

What was Facebook founder Mark Zuckerberg's motto? "Move fast and break things."

We're not "things," but the tech companies are breaking us just the same.

And we are seemingly helpless to stop the next big leap forward, the latest tweak, the hottest tech that will revolutionize everyone's life whether we want it to or not. We're all trapped in a bad sci-fi movie.

As is true everywhere else in the world of Fatal Conveniences, the hazards are especially risky for kids. Unlike adults, they were born into the digital age, meaning they've been exposed to EMR from birth (and even earlier). Their bodies are more vulnerable than ours. Their reproductive systems are the ones that need protection. But they're not getting it.

According to an Environmental Working Group analysis of existing research, radiation from wireless digital sources, including cell phones, can cause changes in sleep habits and increase the risk of dizziness, tremors, headaches, memory difficulties, and behavioral changes, especially in children. It may even be responsible for an increased risk of tumors in the brain and inner ear, including malignancies. There's also evidence to suggest that EMR has serious effects on our nervous systems and our behaviors.

Do you wonder why I'm so scared? And angry? How can we know all that and still go through life acting as though our digital devices are our friends?

Meanwhile, we are sprinting toward ever more electrification. Toward more and more data being transferred wirelessly. Toward more radiation spewing everywhere.

This all reminds me of what we went through with cigarettes. Look back now at our attitudes about smoking in the 1940s, '50s, '60s, and '70s. We thought that smokers were so cool and glamorous.

Smoking kills slowly, over the course of decades. The damage is cumulative. Is radiation—even the nonionizing kind—operating the same way? We can't possibly know, because the technology hasn't been around long enough for us to measure its long-term effects.

Is buying your kid a cell phone, an Apple Watch, or a laptop computer the same thing as giving him or her a pack of smokes and a lighter? Will we find out too late?

We already know many of the ways in which EMR puts our bodies under stress. Testosterone markers go down. Immune system and free-radical damage go up. Cell senescence is distorted, so the natural death cycle of the cells is altered, and cancer rates go up. All this and a whole lot more continues to happen, and we're still not doing anything about it. The smartest people in the world keep their phones in their pants pockets and their bras, their laptops on their laps, up against their most delicate body parts, blasting them with potentially lethal electromagnetic fields.

And no one is taking responsibility. No regulatory body has got your back.

In 2015, the European Commission's Scientific Committee on Emerging and Newly Identified Health Risks reviewed the research on electromagnetic fields in general and cell phones in particular. It found that even extremely-low-frequency EMFs could be linked to an increased risk of childhood leukemia. How did we not all know that? How was that not front-page news? It's interesting what else the committee said: that so far, no studies have determined exactly *how* cell phones might give kids that terrible disease.

What does that tell us? It tells us that nobody with the funding or the expertise to figure it out really wants us to know—because once we know, somebody will have to do something about it. It reminds me of the playbook the tobacco companies used for decades: the old "we're not sure because it needs more testing" and then never actually doing the credible research, just kicking the questions down the road.

Consider this from the *International Journal of Oncology*, published in 2017:

> The [International Agency for Research on Cancer] working group reached the conclusion that RF radiation from devices that emit non-ionizing RF radiation . . . is a Group 2B, i.e. a "possible," human carcinogen. . . .
>
> Several laboratory studies have indicated mechanisms of action for RF radiation carcinogenesis such as on DNA repair, oxidative stress, down regulation of mRNA and DNA damage with single strand breaks. A report was released from The National Toxicology Program (NTP) under the National Institutes of Health (NIH) in the USA on the largest ever animal study on cell phone RF radiation and cancer. An increased incidence of glioma in the brain and malignant schwannoma in the heart was found in rats. Acoustic neuroma or vestibular schwannoma is a similar type of tumour as the one found in the heart, although benign. Thus, this animal study supported human epidemiological findings on RF radiation and brain tumour risk.

The study included all sources of radiation, including mobile phone base stations, Wi-Fi access points, smartphones, laptops, and tablets. The report went on to say, "For children this risk may be accentuated because of a cumulative effect during a long lifetime use. Developing and immature cells can also be more sensitive to exposure to RF radiation."

Sound familiar? One cigarette can't hurt you, but many, over decades, can.

Were you aware of any of those studies? Now that you know, how do you feel about your tech habits and those of your children? Look, I get it—because all the waves and radiation we're discussing in this chapter are invisible, it's easy to pretend they don't exist. Except that they do. The world of consumer tech and digital devices is the ultimate Fatal Convenience. You can easily find nonharmful shampoos, food containers, or any of the other products I've been talking about in this book. But where are you going to find replacements for the technology we depend on day in and out?

Nowhere. It's a serious problem. There *are* solutions. Not enough. But some.

THROUGHOUT THIS BOOK, I'VE TRIED to come up with suggestions for avoiding Fatal Conveniences by seeking out healthy alternatives. After giving you the bad news, I've looked for ways of answering the obvious question: "Okay, so now what do we do?" Even though this chapter's subject matter is tricky and complex, and not totally understood even by the experts, we need to answer the same question: Now what?

No matter which type of digital technology or device we're talking about, the issues are pretty much the same: we're being bathed in electromagnetic radiation, and we're more or less helpless to stop it. But the ways we use each form of technology are different. Here's the main thing to remember: electromagnetic energy is always greatest nearest the source. The greater the distance we can create between our bodies and our gadgets, the better off we'll be. That feels like common sense. It's a useful rule of thumb.

Here's another: wired is better than wireless.

We might never be truly safe. But we can be safer. Let's see how.

FATAL CONVENIENCES: CELL PHONES AND 5G

I admit that cell phones are a miracle. They're magic. I've been lost in countries in the developing world, far from anything or anyone I knew, and they have saved my skin. Cell phones turned the concept of expensive long-distance calls into a dim memory, since "distance" no longer exists, at least as we once understood it. Your voice is turned into an electronic signal that is encoded so it can be bounced off satellites and transmitted via cell towers that can read the signal and send it along to the next cell at the speed of light, 186,000 or so miles per second, and once it reaches your device, you hear something that sounds exactly like me. No wonder we treasure our devices—your cell phone is more important to you than your gallbladder.

The first call ever made from a handheld device was back in 1973, from a device that weighed around two and a half pounds, about half as much as a brick. You had to charge it for ten hours, and then it worked for only thirty minutes of talk time. The first consumer model, the Motorola DynaTAC, cost $3,995, equivalent to $10,420 today. It now seems as though every person in the world owns a cell phone. A little over half of kids in the United States have a smartphone by the time they're eleven, a statistic that really scares me.

Right now, many of us take advantage of the miracle known as 5G connectivity. It has replaced 4G, which replaced 3G, and so on. Thanks to this latest tech, our devices move more data, and faster, than ever before. If you're old enough to remember dial-up internet connections, you know what I'm talking about. (And if you're not, consider yourself lucky.) At some point, 6G, the sixth generation of connectivity, will be here, making our phones and other devices even more amazingly powerful and, yes, convenient.

The thing about 5G, though, is that its high-frequency millimeter waves don't travel as far as its predecessors' did. This means that many more small cell towers have had to be put in place all around us. 5G transmission also burns more energy than that of the Gs that came before. When I travel around my neighborhood today, I see 5G cell stations all over the place: on telephone poles, on top of schools, everywhere. Why does that matter? Because the electrical energy storm that surrounds us, our total immersion in radiation, is bigger and stronger than ever. And we *still* don't know how much damage it's doing to our health. We just know that it's now even more inescapable.

We've already seen some evidence of the risks we run when using cell phones. But there's plenty more. A 2017 review of existing research into phone use and glioma, a type of cancerous tumor found in the brain and nervous system, was conducted by scientists in China. They came to this conclusion: "Our results suggest that long-term mobile phone use may be associated with an increased risk of glioma. There was also an association between mobile phone use and low-grade glioma in the regular use or long-term use subgroups."

But as so often happens, the authors were unable to establish hard proof of a link due to the lack of better studies. Here's what they said: "Current evidence is of poor quality and limited quantity. It is therefore necessary to conduct large sample, high quality research or better characterization of any potential association between long-term ipsilateral mobile phone use and glioma risk."

Two years before that report, the European Commission's Scientific Committee on Emerging and Newly Identified Health Risks reviewed electromagnetic fields in general and cell phones in particular. It found that overall, epidemiologic studies of extremely-low-frequency fields showed an increased risk of childhood leukemia, even though the research couldn't determine exactly what about cell phone use caused it. In other words, we know enough to be scared but not enough to know *how* scared or precisely why. That's the reason we continue to be exposed to potentially carcinogenic radiation.

Cancer isn't the only thing we need to be worried about. The blood-brain barrier is a wall of cells that prevents certain harmful molecules from traveling from your bloodstream into your brain. It's yet another miracle of our bodies. Without it we'd all be dead. What does that have to do with EMR? Albumin, a protein found in the bloodstream, does not normally enter the brain. But when lab rats are exposed to the kind of radiation emitted by cell phones, albumin is detected in their brains—evidence of a breach in the blood-brain barrier.

In 2003, Swedish scientists performed studies on rats to see whether radiation of the kind we get from cell phones caused a breakdown of the blood-brain barrier. Here's what they wrote at the end of their report:

We chose 12–26-week-old rats because they are comparable with human teenagers—notably frequent users of mobile phones—with respect to age. The situation of the growing brain might deserve special concern from society because biologic and maturational processes are particularly vulnerable during the growth process. The intense use of mobile phones by youngsters is a serious consideration. A neuronal damage of the kind described here may not have immediately demonstrable consequences, even if repeated. In the long run, however, it may result in reduced brain reserve capacity that might be unveiled by other later neuronal disease or even the wear and tear of aging. We cannot exclude that after some decades of (often) daily use, a whole generation of users may suffer negative effects, perhaps as early as in middle age.

In a 2006 presentation at a conference on EMF and health, the authors stated that years of cell phone use "may promote the development of autoimmune and neuro-degenerative diseases, and we conclude that the suppliers of mobile communication—and our politicians—have an extensive responsibility to support the exploration of these possible risks for the users and the society."

That was way back in 2006, when the latest technology was 3G. Nearly two decades later, we're still waiting for the mobile communication giants and our political leaders to address these dangers.

Here's yet another terrifying question: Do cell phones damage our ability to produce sperm? In 2021, a review and analysis of cell phone research was published in the scientific journal *Environmental Research*. The researchers looked at more than a hundred studies, and here's what they found: "Mobile phone use decreased the overall sperm quality by affecting the motility, viability, and concentration. It was further reduced in the group with high mobile phone usage. In particular, the decrease was remarkable in *in vivo* studies with stronger clinical significance in subgroup analysis. Therefore, long-term cell phone use is a factor that must be considered as a cause of sperm quality reduction."

In another study, conducted with a group of subjects who had attended infertility clinics, the men who used their phones most often or kept their phones in their pockets produced less sperm than the rest of the participants. This, the study's authors said, "might support the suggestion of the negative effect of prolonged cell phone use on male fertility."

In a 2016 survey of existing research, sperm damage was found in twenty-one of twenty-seven studies reviewed. Speaking of reproductive hazards, a 2017 study showed that low-frequency magnetic fields can even increase the risk of miscarriage.

Research done at the Cleveland Clinic looked at cell phone use among men and whether it affected their sperm in any meaningful way. Here's what they found: the more time men spent on their phones, the more damage their sperm sustained. Everything—sperm count, motility, and viability—went down. The subjects were four groups of males: Group 1, not using phones at all; Group 2, using them two hours a day; Group 3, using them two to four hours daily; and Group 4, using them more than four hours a day. You know what they found? Sperm count was negatively affected as phone use increased! Basically, their phones were neutering them. Now think of the exposure your kids are getting. Clearly, there's a need for more research into what exactly is going on here.

It seems as though there are never enough credible studies, never sufficient scientific evidence, to prove what many people (me included) already believe: that we're endangering our health by absorbing so much radiation.

My frustrating search for hard-core proof went on and on until just about the time I was finishing this chapter. That was when I found it: the first research I've seen to prove beyond the shadow of a doubt that 5G definitely harms our health, by causing something called "the microwave syndrome."

The article was published in 2022 in the Swedish journal *Medicinsk Access*, based on a study conducted by Lennart Hardell, a Swedish oncologist and researcher from the Forskningsstiftelsen Miljö & Cancer (Research Foundation for Environment & Cancer), and Mona Nilsson from the Strålskyddsstiftelsen (Radiation Protection Foundation). They looked at what happened after a 5G base station was installed on the roof of an apartment building, just five meters above one unit's bedroom. Measurements taken before and after the installation showed what the study called a massive increase in radiation in the apartment. Previously, there had been base stations for 3G and 4G in the same place, but once they were exchanged for 5G, the radiation level nearly doubled.

According to the study, the couple living in the apartment immediately began to suffer from a long list of symptoms, including fatigue, difficulty sleeping, nosebleeds, tinnitus, skin problems, dizziness, concentration problems, and heart palpitations—all of which decreased or disappeared within a day after they moved to another home with significantly lower radiation. All the conditions they suffered under exposure to 5G radio waves are identical to those first described more than fifty years ago by people who received whole-body microwave radiation.

That's only one study, I realize. I wish there were a thousand more out there. But it's enough for me. It proves that despite what the telecommunications spokespeople and other so-called experts want us to believe, the radiation that's all around us thanks to our cell phones and other wireless devices is harmful to our health. How harmful? We don't know. That's what makes it so hard to evaluate.

Do I take advantage of 5G? Of course I do. However, I'd like it a whole lot more if it used fiber-optic lines to carry the data and the lines were buried underground. Instead, those little cell stations are everywhere, bathing us all in who knows what.

As connectivity gets faster, better, and smoother, our reliance on our phones will grow. Meaning we'll be using them even more than we do now, exposing ourselves to . . . what?

KNOWING ALL THAT, WHAT SHOULD we do? Here's the number one thing: never, but never, hold your phone against your ear and talk. To me, holding a cell phone against your head during a conversation is as bad as smoking cigarettes—or worse. When we use a cell phone that way, we're increasing our risk of developing tumors of the brain and inner ear, possibly even malignancies.

Kids today almost never talk on their phones—they'd rather text, which is smart because it cuts down on the exposure of their brains and auditory nerves to radiation.

If you must talk on your phone, do it with wired headphones plus a microphone. Even better, get antiradiation air tube headphones. My friends at Tech Wellness (techwellness.com) make good ones. Certainly, don't use wireless Bluetooth earbuds. Anything that creates distance between your body parts and your phone is a good thing. The same goes for anything else that doesn't require a Bluetooth connection.

Remember: Wires are good!

The Environmental Working Group has sensible advice for how to use a cell phone:

+ Use it as little as possible. Don't carry it with you constantly; put it away until you need it. It's a tool, not a toy.
+ When you're not using it, put it into airplane mode, so it emits no pulsed radiation due to the phone's always trying to connect. Turn it off at night. Whatever you do, don't sleep with your phone near your head or next to your body. I recently saw a study saying that three-quarters of young people sleep with their phones under their pillows. That's a *really* bad idea.
+ Boys and men, do not carry your phone in a front pants pocket. Keeping it out of every pocket is even smarter. Considering all the evidence that EMR can alter hormones and damage both sperm quality *and* quantity, this is a must. You might want to have a kid someday.
+ Girls and women, don't ever put your phone into your bra or into a breast or back pocket. We're still guessing about the power of radiation to cause cancer. The safest bet is to carry it in your bag or backpack—anywhere but next to your body.

To all that, I'll add these tips:

+ Use speaker mode when you must talk.
+ Avoid making calls when the signal is weak, as this causes your phone to boost its radio frequency (RF) transmission power.
+ Consider sending voice memos, my own favorite method of communication.

Not every phone emits an equal amount of radiation. The specific absorption rate (SAR) is the amount of RF energy from a given phone that is absorbed by the user's body. Different cell phones have different SAR levels. Cell phone makers are required to report the maximum SAR level of their products to the FCC. This information can often be found on the manufacturer's website or in the phone's user manual. The upper limit of SAR allowed in the United States according to FCC safety guidelines is 1.6 watts per kilogram (W/kg) of body weight.

But comparing the SAR values of phones can be misleading. The listed value is based only on the phone operating at its highest power, not on what users would typically be exposed to with normal use. The actual SAR during use varies based on a number of factors, so it's possible that a phone with a lower SAR value might expose a person to more RF waves than one with a higher SAR value.

Keep in mind that even when you're not using your phone, it is constantly looking for a signal and therefore is always emitting radiation.

Here's something else you can do: Buy a protective device for your phone, such as Safe Sleeve (safesleevecases.com), which can block more than 99 percent of radio frequency, or RF (5G, Wi-Fi, cellular, etc.), and 92 percent of extremely-low-frequency, or ELF (battery, AC power, etc.), radiation.

Or try Waveguard (waveguard.com). My good buddy and company founder Hagen Thiers was sensitive to EMR as a kid, and his father set out to help him solve the problem. They came up with this amazing piece of tech. I am a fan of the company's devices because they decrease stress on the body and still allow us to enjoy the benefits of Wi-Fi and cell phones. The company's website includes information from several studies, including one on how cell phone radiation impairs how well wounds heal. Pretty amazing stuff.

Tech Wellness (techwellness.com) is another great resource. August Brice posts a lot of information about her products, including Ethernet cables that allow you to switch your phone to airplane mode and then, using their adapter, plug the ethernet cable into your phone.

Here's one final thing we can all do: reach out to Elon Musk and tell him not to put nearly forty thousand satellites into the atmosphere to blanket the earth with 5G and other forms of EMR. Come on, Elon! We need you to gather more safety data before we allow you and other tech companies to reap profits at the expense of our safety.

FATAL CONVENIENCES: WI-FI AND ROUTERS

Here's two more Fatal Conveniences with a backstory.

Most people remember Hedy Lamarr as an Austrian-born Hollywood movie star from back in the 1930s, a total femme fatale. But she also invented a technology used to prevent enemy ships from jamming our torpedo guidance systems. She and her coinventor, a composer named George Antheil, found a way for the radio-operated systems that guided our torpedoes to jump from one frequency to another, thereby making it impossible for an enemy to block the message. Their invention became known as "frequency hopping" and was a big help to the Allied naval forces.

For years afterward, the technology found further uses, first in telecommunications and then in an innovation officially known as IEEE 802.11b, or, a little easier to remember, "wireless fidelity," or Wi-Fi. So thank Hedy and George for the fact that your router can direct data from the internet to the various devices in your home, school, and office.

Is there anything else our routers give us? The same kind of radiation emitted by all other wireless devices. According to the "experts," our routers are not dangerous at all. At the same time, however, we're advised to keep our distance from them. Hmm . . .

We need to be especially careful not to position routers too close to where children sleep or play. But we can take stronger measures, too. Since not using a router would also mean we'd not have access to Wi-Fi, getting rid of it is a nonstarter. Short of throwing away your cell phone, it would probably be the most drastic antitech step we could take.

I'm sure there's at least one generation of human beings who can't even remember a time before Wi-Fi existed. For them—really, for most of us—it's like oxygen: invisible, everywhere, and necessary to life.

So what should you do instead? Connect your computer to your modem with an old-school Ethernet cable. That's the easiest solution. Or you could put your router on a timer so it automatically turns off at night. But you could also consider using a Faraday cage or a router shield.

Michael Faraday was an English genius and practical science pioneer who invented the first electric motor dynamo, produced the first electrical current from a magnetic field, and essentially set the stage for electromagnetic field theory. He did all that during the nineteenth century, but his name has been co-opted for a number of current-day tech innovations, such as Faraday bicycles, to name just one. Another is the Faraday cage, which is a fairly simple thing—a mesh metal box that goes over your router and blocks it from emitting some (but not all) of its radiation. This technology was originally designed to limit interference and noise from magnetic and electric fields so correct scientific measurements could be taken.

Today you can buy not just a cage to go over your router but also small bags to hold your phone, enabling it to send or receive messages or calls.

There are plenty of products that claim to protect us from EMR. Many are junk with no scientific data to support them—like weird stickers to put on your phone, expensive pendants, or underwear. But others truly work.

FATAL CONVENIENCE: BLUETOOTH

The tenth-century Danish king Harald Gormsson supposedly had a dead tooth that turned blue-gray, which led to his colorful nickname: Bluetooth. He was also famous for uniting Scandinavia, which was why his name was chosen—originally only as a placeholder—until a proper one could be found by the combine of Nokia, Intel, and Ericsson for the short-range wireless connection technology they developed.

The name Bluetooth stuck, and it's now everywhere, literally—all around us, connecting everything, emitting radiation everywhere it goes. By now the list of devices depending on Bluetooth is endless and keeps getting longer, meaning we're constantly filling the atmosphere with more radiation. That's the main thing to keep in mind, especially if you're concerned—as you should be—about how all that radiation is affecting your health.

Just think: Fitbits, smart watches, video game controllers, Google glasses, home thermostats, VR headsets, video sunglasses, your car, your refrigerator, your headphones, your sex toys, and a whole lot more, plus all those body function monitors that track your REM sleep, perform EKGs and automatically send the results to your online medical record, and measure your blood pressure, respiration, and any other bodily function that can be observed, quantified, and stored somewhere.

It's the so-called Internet of Things—except that "things" now includes you and me.

Insider Intelligence forecasts 3.74 billion mobile connections worldwide by 2025 and more than 64 billion connected devices by 2026. What does that mean for us? Lots more radiation flying around, creating an even bigger, broader electromagnetic field for us to inhabit whether we want to or not. How harmful is all that?

It could be worse. Bluetooth headphone exposures fall anywhere between one-tenth and one-four-hundredth what we get from our cell phones, according to the Dana-Farber Cancer Institute's Dr. David Kozono. "I would therefore expect it would be more difficult to observe an association between Bluetooth headphone use and cancer," he said. But then he added, "Data are lacking however to conclude with certainty that there is or is not a risk of increased cancer."

See what I mean? We're the guinea pigs in somebody's real-world lab experiments.

Consumer Reports has done a terrific job of reporting on this stuff. Its staff interviewed Jerry Phillips, a professor of biochemistry at the University of Colorado, Colorado Springs, who said that research has yet to determine how low radiation has to be before it can be considered harmless. They also spoke with David Carpenter, a physician and director of the Institute for Health and the Environment at the University at Albany–State University of New York. He said that being near a single router might be harmless, but often we're in the presence of many computers and routers, as in schools and apartment buildings.

In 2016, the Maryland State Department of Education recommended that schools use wired networks instead of Wi-Fi, turn off routers when not being used, and keep them as far as possible from kids. France has banned Wi-Fi from nursery schools. Now, that is a good idea!

For household appliances and other devices used in the home that require electricity, magnetic field levels are highest near the source of the field and decrease rapidly the farther away the user is from the source. Magnetic fields drop big time at a distance of about one foot from most appliances. For computer screens, at a distance of twelve to twenty inches levels are similarly lower.

FATAL CONVENIENCES: MICROWAVE OVENS

This is the kitchen convenience that seemed like magic when it was introduced back in the 1960s. Suddenly, food that took what felt like forever to cook or reheat came out of this high-tech box in a few minutes and was hotter than hell. We had no idea how exactly it worked—most of us still don't—but it did the job better than anything else we could imagine, so it was okay by us. Today, close to 100 percent of American homes have one, and we use them often.

They have a suitably sci-fi backstory. In 1946, a Raytheon engineer was trying to boost the power level of magnetron tubes used in radar when he accidentally discovered the waves' heating capability. It took another twenty years for Amana's famous Radarange to invade America's kitchens. Microwave ovens work by blasting microwaves, which are a little shorter than radio waves, causing the water molecules in the food inside the oven to vibrate at a high frequency, which in turn heats the food. That's why liquids and vegetables that contain a lot of water heat so fast. There's no actual warming involved, just a lot of very excited molecules.

Of course, that's what makes microwaves so scary: there's a chamber full of radiation sitting on your kitchen counter! But because the radiation is nonionizing, it has no power to break up atoms and so has no effect on our bodies (or so we're told). The potential for danger would be if the oven's casing gets damaged, and supposedly that doesn't happen with normal use. In fact, FDA rules require that microwave ovens be designed to prevent radiation leaks.

Assuming that the oven itself is safe, how about the food? Does cooking it in a microwave rob it of nutritional value or in any way make it dangerous to eat? All cooking causes vitamins to break down, and when we boil vegetables in water, some nutrition is lost. But because microwaves cook so quickly and without water, they actually preserve some of the beneficial molecules our food contains.

Still, my instincts tell me that microwave ovens are bad news. They're messing with the internal molecular structure of the food we eat. To me, that sounds like it could backfire on us. There are ways to cook and reheat our food without blasting it with radiation. Maybe your stovetop or toaster oven will take a little longer to do the job. I'm willing to wait a minute or two extra if it means I can leave the molecules of my dinner unmolested.

How About the Environment?

As far as I'm concerned, radiation is a form of air pollution, maybe even worse than what vehicles or smokestacks spew into our lungs. But the environmental impact of the digital world goes well beyond that. There's a growing body of research on how radiation affects wildlife and insects such as bees and butterflies. One study from 2018 suggested that EMFs emitted by power lines may stress out honeybees and potentially mess with their ability to pollinate crops—our food!

A study by researchers at McMaster University published in the *Journal of Cleaner Production* analyzed the carbon impact of the entire information and communications technology (ICT) industry from around 2010 to 2020, including personal computers, laptops, monitors, smartphones, and servers. Here's what the researchers found: that even as our devices have become more energy efficient, the overall environmental impact of technology is getting worse. ICT produced 1 percent of the global carbon footprint in 2007. Today that figure has nearly tripled and is on its way to exceed 14 percent by 2040. That's half as much as the entire transportation industry.

Okay, So Now What Should We Do?

Besides the precautions I've mentioned above, I've hard wired everything possible in my home. I'm plugged back in. I'm swimming against the tide, I realize. The world is becoming more connected wirelessly day by day. Every smart appliance, every wearable, produces more radiation. Just because you can't see it doesn't mean it's not there.

Researchers look at our electronic devices individually and pronounce that none of them endangers our health. But we aren't exposed to only our phones or only our laptops. We're hit with radiation from multiple sources all at once, all the time. It's the same phenomenon as with all the industrial chemicals that pound us day after day; it's not one thing that's doing the damage, it's *everything*.

I know I've said this before, but it's like that poor camel's back: it took just one straw too many to break it. I'm not focusing on one source of radiation or one new technology. I'm looking at the physical stress caused by *all* of them. That's not what I want in my life.

How about you?

7

CLOTHING

FOR PRACTICALLY MY ENTIRE ADULT LIFE, I've been superaware and super-careful about what I put on my skin. Like I said earlier, my father's experience with chemical sensitivity opened my eyes to the harmful toxins contained in ordinary consumer products. So I've done my best to avoid each and every nasty one.

But it never occurred to me that something just as bad was rubbing against nearly every inch of me almost twenty-four hours a day: my clothes!

My eyes were opened when I met Jeff Garner, an artist who also designs a line of sustainable, healthy, truly beautiful fashions under the name Prophetik. His creations have been worn to the Academy Awards and appeared in *Vogue*, so he's the real thing. He mentioned to me that everything he makes is colored using vegetable dyes only. When I asked him if chemical tints were truly so bad, Jeff was like, "Dude, your clothes are spewing formaldehyde at you! They're off-gassing all kinds of gnarly stuff." That's what started me down the path of examining how our clothing is made and why it harms us.

It wasn't always this way. In the beginning, clothes were made of natural fibers only: wool, cotton, linen, hemp, silk, hides, fur. The raw materials didn't need much in the way of processing. When textiles were tinted, nature's own dyes were used. They did the job.

They still do; soak a clean white T-shirt in hot water with a raw beet in it for red or some powdered turmeric for yellow, and see for yourself. I've done this myself: a vest I really like got stained, so I put it into hot water along with some powdered chaga mushrooms, and it came out dark brown—and stain free. Way back in time, we also made dyes from minerals and even insects. And that was about it.

Fabrics today are treated with a long list of man-made chemicals and synthetic dyes plus a whole lot more. We buy garments that we never need to iron because they're "permanent press," "no-iron," or "wrinkle free." Our clothing boasts that it's stain resistant, waterproof, flame retardant, oil resistant, odor fighting, even antimicrobial.

Where do you think all those extra features—those superpowers— come from? Textiles are manufactured and treated with industrial-strength chemicals, many of which aren't tested before they're put into use. Some contain toxic substances proven by research to cause harm to living things. Some are known carcinogens.

What about the long list of nonnatural fabrics, everything from polyester, nylon, and fleece to spandex and Lycra? They all require little care, they're usually cheaper than natural textiles, and they wear really well. Sweatsuits and yoga pants, which once were worn only in the gym or on the track, now show up everywhere. They're made of high-tech, cool-looking fabrics.

But they're all petroleum based—made from oil—and engineered in corporate labs. Many fabrics contain tiny particles of metal or plastic microbeads, which are shed every time we wear them or wash them. They wind up on our skin, in our lungs, in waterways, in aquatic plant and animal life; they are even found in the water used to irrigate farm crops. In a way, what's happened to clothing is just like what's changed about our food supply: once it was all natural, and today it's ultraprocessed— transformed into industrial products without a lot of concern about how that will affect our health.

When we get dressed, we think we know what we're putting on, but in reality, we have no idea. We're careful about what we allow inside our bodies, but somehow we forget that our skin is a vital organ that's exposed virtually twenty-four hours a day to the clothing we wear. Skin's main job is to protect us from the external world, so maybe we figure that nothing bad can get through.

But that isn't the case; our skin is permeable. Things that touch us on the surface can shed substances that make their way inside to our bloodstream and from there to all other parts of our bodies. We're all familiar with how patches are placed on the skin to transport medications to our internal organs. We may not want to think that harmful chemicals can get inside the same way. But they can, and they do.

Here's a good example. In 2016, some flight attendants on American Airlines were issued new uniforms. The attendants immediately began experiencing weird phenomena, everything from rashes, hives, and headaches to bloody noses, respiratory difficulties, and autoimmune disease symptoms. Some of them ended up hospitalized. In all, five thousand airline employees reported problems once they began wearing the new outfits.

Even passengers on their flights were affected; a baby held just for a moment by one attendant developed a rash, which was attributed to the chemicals used in manufacturing the uniform fabrics. That's an extreme case, granted. But I guarantee you that the same toxic chemicals that caused those reactions are in the clothing we all wear every day. They contain the same likely carcinogens, the same caustic irritants. We're all being inundated with them, in most cases not at levels high enough to make us noticeably sick. Not yet.

In this chapter, I'll talk about the harm we suffer and the risks we run from wearing the things we wear. But I'll also get into the less obvious health hazards: the huge environmental toll that comes from the way our clothes are made.

You don't have to take my word about our clothing's impact on the planet. This is from a 2019 report prepared by the British Parliament's House of Commons Environmental Audit Committee, titled *Fixing Fashion: Clothing Consumption and Sustainability*:

The way we make, use and throwaway our clothes is unsustainable. Textile production contributes more to climate change than international aviation and shipping combined, consumes lake-sized volumes of fresh water and creates chemical and plastic pollution. Synthetic fibres are being found in the deep sea, in Arctic sea ice, in fish and shellfish. Our biggest retailers have "chased the cheap needle around the planet," commissioning production in countries with low pay, little trade union representation and weak environmental protection. In many countries, poverty pay and conditions are standard for garment workers, most of whom are women. We are also concerned about the use of child labour, prison labour, forced labour and bonded labour in factories and the garment supply chain. Fast fashions' overproduction and overconsumption of clothing is based on the globalisation of indifference towards these manual workers.

The damage the production of our clothes does to the environment is enormous. Huge volumes of water are used in textile dyeing, along with comparable amounts of energy. Dyeing cotton requires 125 liters of water per kilogram of fabric; meaning that the manufacture of a single T-shirt uses fifteen to twenty liters of water. Globally, the textile industry uses 21 trillion liters of water annually and is responsible for an estimated one-fifth of all industrial water pollution. That's because of all the dyes, salts, heavy metals, and other chemicals used, which form a toxic soup.

The World Bank tested sample waterways in locations where textiles are manufactured and found seventy-two dangerous chemicals. Once the dyes are released into rivers and streams, they form a tinted film that blocks out light, killing animal and plant life. These chemicals then make their way from the water into the food chain, where they can be found in vegetables and fruits.

Maybe the most dangerous thing about clothing is that it doesn't seem like an environmental hazard. When you see a photo of thousands of plastic bags floating around in the middle of the ocean or empty water bottles desecrating a beautiful riverbank, or watch a video of sea animals being choked to death by plastic six-pack rings, you're horrified by the obscenity of all that toxic trash.

But our clothes? They look so comfortable and familiar. What could be the harm in a nice, soft cotton T-shirt? Or some cool new jeans?

Plenty, it turns out. Think of all the T-shirts and jeans there are in the world—in your clothes closet, in every apparel store, on every fashion e-commerce website.

Everything we wear creates an environmental impact—from farming to manufacturing, even to laundering. For the most part, fabrics are made and turned into garments in poor countries for the simple reason that labor costs there are disgracefully low. We might be tempted to believe that the pollution from manufacturing, preparing, treating, and dyeing textiles and turning them into apparel poisons only those parts of the planet.

Think again.

First, we all live in the same world; when we defile it, every part gets defiled. This dynamic comes up time and again when we discuss our consumer habits—there's literally no distance between ourselves and the environmental damage our Fatal Conveniences cause. It all comes home. I've said this repeatedly throughout the book, mainly because it's so easy for us to forget or ignore that all our consumer choices come with a cost—to the health of the planet as well as our own.

You may not be aware that your new jeans contain microscopic plastic beads. When you wash them, they go from your washer into the water supply and before long right back into you. They're in the air we breathe and the food we eat. And how about the pesticides and other harsh chemicals used to grow and dye cotton, hemp, and other plant fibers? And the petrochemicals used to make polyester, nylon, and other synthetic fabrics? Today, the majority of clothing sold in the world is made of nonnatural materials, mainly petroleum based. In addition to the carbon footprint of that unsustainable source of fabric, factor in the industrial processes required to turn oil into clothing. Don't forget the cruel, environmentally devastating animal slaughter needed to produce leather and suede shoes, outerwear, and other clothing.

What makes things even worse is the huge amount of waste in the system. By one estimate, more than 15 million tons of textiles are wasted annually—never used in products, gone instead straight into landfills. An outfit called Reverse Resources hosts an online marketplace that connects fabric factories and fashion designers who want to use leftover material to make clothes. According to a 2016 study, the garment industry creates almost enough wasted textiles annually to cover the entire country of Estonia.

Now, maybe you're not a geography wizard, so you don't know how big Estonia is: 17,463 square miles. That means we're talking about a lot of wasted fabric, along with all the resources used to create it. Globally, according to estimates, roughly one-third of all food is wasted somewhere along the line from producers to consumers, and now we're seeing the same level of heedless, destructive waste when it comes to fabric and apparel. Squandering resources seems to be built into the way we humans operate, but it doesn't have to be that way. These are massively failed and failing systems!

Regeneration (regeneration.org), founded by my buddy Paul Hawken, is a force for good when it comes to the way our consumer habits interact with the environment and our health. Its website is packed with information and useful ideas about how we can become better, smarter clothing buyers. Here are a few of its suggestions:

- **Wash your clothing less often.** This keeps pollutants such as plastic and other substances out of the water supply. It also means that your clothes will last longer. And there are devices made for use in our washing machines that capture shed plastic microparticles before they can be released into the water supply.
- **Repair and recycle.** Next time a T-shirt gets a hole in it, don't throw it away; turn it into something else, something unique and cool, or

cover the hole with a patch. Back in the 1960s, people paved over the holes in their worn jeans with all kinds of groovy patches. We thought it made our clothes even cooler. Or maybe your dog needs a T-shirt.

+ **Trade with your friends.** This is another trend young consumers are adopting: when you've either outgrown garments or become bored with them, call some buddies over and offer to swap with clothing they're ready to get rid of. You can get a whole new wardrobe this way for zero dollars and no environmental impact.

+ **Sell your used clothes.** Today, on online marketplaces such as The RealReal (therealreal.com), you can make money from your good-quality used clothing, especially things that cost a lot and are still in style.

+ **Give your old clothes away.** Nonprofits such as Goodwill and Salvation Army have been recycling clothing since long before it was trendy.

As you can see, there's a lot here to think about. Let's get started.

FATAL CONVENIENCES: STAIN-RESISTANT, WATERPROOF, WRINKLE-FREE CLOTHING

It takes work to keep our clothes looking good. After we wash them, we have to iron them, because who wants wrinkles? Once we're wearing them, we try to keep them clean and neat and looking sharp. So it was probably only a matter of time before science came to the rescue. Next thing you know, we're wearing clothes that practically take care of themselves: no more ironing; no more stains; clothes that refuse to get wet.

But there must be a price to pay; there's always a price. In this case, it's the industrial-strength toxicity that comes with those conveniences.

I discussed this earlier: the PFAS group of chemicals. A brief recap: they started life as Teflon and Scotchgard, and their main function is to make things slippery. That's why stains and oil don't stick to treated clothes and water runs off without soaking in. They're kind of miracle substances—until you realize some of their unadvertised features.

PFASs, as I've said before, are known as "forever chemicals," meaning that instead of breaking down they build up, both in the environment and inside our bodies (this is called *bioaccumulation*). They can do us serious harm: according to the International Agency for Research on Cancer, part of the World Health Organization, PFASs are "likely carcinogenic" and have been associated with:

- Kidney cancer
- Testicular cancer
- Liver disease
- Ulcerative colitis
- Thyroid problems
- Decreased birth weight
- High cholesterol
- Neurotoxicity
- Immune system dysfunction
- Hormone disruption

That's an unbelievable list of horrible effects these chemicals can have on us, isn't it? In addition, children, because of their size and developing immune systems, are even more susceptible to PFAS toxicity. According to one study, exposure to the chemicals caused a 50 percent decrease in antibody concentration in children aged five to seven.

Aside from wearing them, we're constantly being exposed to PFASs in the environment; as we've already seen, these chemicals are in a long list of consumer products from dental floss and fast-food burger wrappers to electronic components and cosmetics—literally thousands of things we all come into contact with each and every day. By now the chemicals are so widely dispersed in the environment that they've contaminated the sources of tap water that serve nearly every American, and an estimated 98 percent of us have PFASs in our bodies. They're inescapable.

That's a good reason to avoid exposing ourselves to them whenever possible, like in our wardrobes. In some cases, that should be easy—believe it or not, there are garments that actually brag about their Teflon content. So read the labels! Waterproof Gore-Tex garments, including shoes and boots, for example, contain Teflon. So don't wear those. But you won't find PFAS listed on clothes' content labels. That's why it's important to avoid wearing *any* garments with superpowers, anything that calls itself stain or oil resistant or waterproof.

The same goes for no-iron, wrinkle-free, permanent press clothing. That superpower is due to the fact that the fabrics are treated with formaldehyde, the chemical normally associated with embalming fluid. But according to the EPA, the WHO, and several other US and international health agencies, it can cause cancer in those of us who are not dead yet. In one lab experiment, even weak concentrations of formaldehyde, when dissolved in simulated human sweat, increased the proliferation of malignant melanoma cells. You read that right: these chemicals, interacting with sweat, increase the risk of developing melanoma.

Formaldehyde can also cause an allergic reaction, called *contact dermatitis*, just by lying against the skin. According to a 2010 Government Accountability Office report to Congress, "contact dermatitis affects the immune system and produces reactions characterized by rashes, blisters, and flaky, dry skin that can itch or burn." You'll never find the word *formaldehyde* on a clothing label. So maybe we should just learn how to iron our clothes (or live with wrinkles).

How About the Environment?

The EPA and several states are taking steps to decrease the amount of PFASs in consumer products. But since these chemicals have lengthy half-lives, they'll be around us for a long, long time no matter what we do today. They are everywhere in our waterways, meaning that they contaminate the animal and plant life there, too.

Okay, So What Should We Do?

Once upon a time, seafaring men wore clothes made of canvas or cotton coated with wax, linseed oil, or tar to keep water out. Eventually the coating rotted and wore off, but at least they didn't damage the planet. Believe it or not, it's still possible to find all-weather clothing that's treated with wax to keep out water. Sometimes it even comes with extra wax so you can keep it moisture proof. Barring that, we just can just refuse to wear clothing that's been treated to give it any of the superpowers discussed here. As I said, there's no mystery involved; the manufacturers boast on the label about all the Fatal Conveniences contained in their clothing. If we buy natural fabrics only and organic whenever possible, we'll cut out a lot of the guesswork. Beyond that, we can try not to stain our clothes with food or anything else, take along dry socks when we go hiking, and buy and use an iron and ironing board—because there *are* no practical, nontoxic alternatives for making clothing that stays dry, resists stains, or refuses to wrinkle.

FATAL CONVENIENCE: JEANS

Of course you look amazing in your tight skinny jeans. If you didn't, you wouldn't wear them, right? They've been going into and out of style for a long time now—once, fashion victims had to lie down on their beds and suck in their bellies to zip up their skin-tight jeans. Then somebody got the brilliant idea to make denim, which had always been a down-home all-cotton fabric, with rubbery elastane (the generic term for Lycra) fibers mixed in, and voilà! stretch denim, which makes your jeans fit better than ever (meaning tighter, naturally). Excellent! Except for the potential downsides, all of which have been linked to too-tight pants, including:

- Urinary tract infections (due to buildup of bacteria thanks to moisture being unable to escape)

+ Vaginosis (ditto)
+ Yeast infections (ditto)
+ Candidiasis (a fungal infection of the vagina)
+ Rashes (due to friction)
+ Low sperm count (caused by excessive heat on the testicles)
+ Loss of blood flow due to testicular torsion (just what it sounds like)
+ Acid reflux, abdominal cramps, even meralgia paresthetica, a painful nerve condition afflicting the legs, all caused by clothing-induced lower body compression

It's not just the young and chic who suffer. Middle-aged and older men who reported abdominal distress radiating into their chests, along with unexplained heartburn, were wearing trousers that were too snug. Dr. Octavio Bessa, Jr., saw enough such patients over twenty years to have named the disorder "tight pants syndrome" in an article published in 1993. How did he diagnose it? Simply by measuring patients' waists and then the waistband of their jeans.

Aren't there safer ways of showing the world what a nice butt you have?

How About the Environment?

Jeans have a natural, wholesome, down-to-earth vibe, but from an environmental point of view they're exactly the opposite. Denim is disastrous partly because it's so popular—around 450 million pairs of jeans are sold annually in the United States alone. Cotton is a notoriously wasteful and damaging crop, due to the pesticides and GMOs that are used on it. And it takes 3,781 liters of water to make *one pair* of jeans. There's a terrific 2017 documentary about fashion's pollution of the world's waterways called *River Blue*. In the opening scene, deep magenta wastewater from a factory spills into a river as the Roman designer and environmental activist Orsola de Castro says, "There is a joke in China that you can tell the 'it' color of the season by looking at the color of the rivers." There's actually a photo taken by NASA of China's Pearl River showing a dark blue streak running right through it.

Even after your jeans have been manufactured, they don't stop polluting. Why do you think the colors fade? Every time we wash our jeans, they release, on average, fifty-six thousand microfibers, nearly invisible strands of material, including microplastics from synthetic textiles, that end up in rivers, the ocean, and elsewhere in the environment. These tiny pieces of your jeans are becoming one of the most prevalent sources of ocean pollution. According to one study conducted by researchers at the University of Toronto, somewhere around one-quarter of all microfibers found in water samples were blue denim. The fibers are found inside fish, so at some point they wind up inside us, too. Scientists even began noticing indigo-colored particles in the Arctic Circle and determined that they had come from denim; that's how well traveled your jeans are.

Okay, So What Should We Do?

First, if you're like the average person and already own seven pairs of jeans, you probably don't need any more. You have better things to do with your money. Second, don't buy pants that strangle you below the waist. Give your genitals a little breathing room. Third, buy vintage/used/preowned jeans rather than new. They shed less fiber and dye in the wash, and you won't be adding to new-denim demand.

Go online and educate yourself a little about environmentally friendly jeans, ones made with organic cotton and natural dyes. Now even big companies such as Levi's are selling used or recycled denim pants and jackets. The company Nudie Jeans tries hard to make denim as green as it is blue—by recycling, reusing, repairing, and so on. But don't stop there; environmentally sensitive denim can be found all over the internet.

I recently met a guy named Alberto Candiani in a regenerative cotton field forty-five minutes from my home in California, where he was working with the Rodale Institute. Alberto comes from generations of Italian denim suppliers. Believe me, he knows the truth and is now developing a healthy alternative to stretch denim with a 100 percent plant-based, compostable product that will replace elastane. Amazing! I hear about stuff like this all the time, and it gives me hope.

A final suggestion: invest in a washing machine filter, which connects to the discharge hose and captures more than 80 percent of microfibers.

FATAL CONVENIENCE: POLYESTER

Polyester is a totally synthetic petroleum-based plastic, full of toxic chemicals but manufactured to look and feel like cloth—and we wear it on our 100 percent natural skin. Do you see how there might be a problem?

Polyester and the other man-made textiles (nylon, acrylic, spandex) are created not just with petroleum but also with acids plus alcohol plus a bunch of other dangerous substances. Sometimes, even coal is used in their manufacture. Each of these, individually, is harmful to the human body. In some cases, they're carcinogenic. In polyester, all of them are combined. Stop and think a second: We're wearing clothes made of oil!

Are we nuts?

We're dressing our children in it, too! Doesn't that make you the least bit worried? It scares the hell out of me.

The components of polyester and other synthetics are mixed to form a compound known as *monomer* or *ester*. This chemical reaction is known as *polymerization* (hence the name *polyester*). The material created during polymerization is extruded while hot into long, extremely strong fibers.

It's no surprise that polyester and other man-made fabrics now outsell cotton and all other natural fibers. As the Council of Fashion Designers of America points out, "Benefits of polyester include durability, versatility, good sunlight resistance, light weight, resistance to wrinkles, resistance to stains, and quick drying time." It's hard to argue with that—and the council didn't even mention the fact that it's extremely cheap to produce. Polyester is largely responsible for the "fast fashion" explosion of a few years ago that churned out so many low-priced, flimsy garments and did such enormous damage to the environment.

The damage isn't just from wearing polyester. When you heat it, as in your clothes dryer, it off-gasses the chemicals it contains, spewing them onto the rest of your clothing and, once you open the dryer door, into the air you and your family breathe. Even your body heat releases polyester's chemicals onto your skin.

A study was done of the effects of polyester underwear on male fertility and found that it not only reduced sperm production and motility but even reduced sexual desire! The reason? What the researchers called "electrostatic potentials" created by the fabric. Is that what you want next to your testicles? Maybe you don't wear synthetic underwear, but the lesson is that polyester clothing can do a lot of invisible damage to a human being. There's even a skin condition called *polyester allergy*, a form of contact dermatitis caused by the chemicals used in making the fabric.

Polyester also shows up in everything from upholstery to mattresses to baby bibs (it's easier to clean than natural fabrics) to auto safety belts, carpeting, and practically anything else made of cloth. Remember, because it's cheap compared to natural fibers, manufacturers use it eagerly.

How About the Environment?

We think of cars and trucks as gas guzzlers that poison the air and support the petroleum industry's trashing of the planet, but think again—our fashion habits also play a big part. Nearly 70 million barrels of oil are used annually to make synthetic textiles—11 million tons of polyester a year and an estimated half-million tons of plastic microfibers are shed into the oceans annually during the washing of polyester, nylon, and the rest. The polyester garments we discard end up in landfills, where they will take more than two hundred years to break down. If you threw away your polyester leisure suit from the 1970s, it's going to be around for a couple of centuries. Maybe by then disco will be back.

Think of every cheap, flimsy Halloween costume you've ever seen (or worn). What do you think they were made of? Imagine the huge dump of toxic costumes every November 1!

Okay, So What Should We Do?

Obviously, the best choice is to avoid all man-made fabrics. Done!

If that's impractical, you can stick with ethical versions, meaning re-cycled. Patagonia began using fabric made from plastic soda bottles back in the 1990s. Parley for the Oceans created Ocean Plastic, materials for the sports, fashion, and luxury industries made of intercepted and up-cycled marine plastic debris. (It also creates informative and beautiful video content, which can be found on its YouTube channel.) And Amur uses recycled polyester to create high-end evening wear.

There are also some cool young designers who take leftover fabric from big apparel manufacturers—wasted material that would otherwise end up in landfills—and turn it into garments. That's good news. Fashion industry "upcycling" also repurposes used fabric and even remakes old clothes. Still, it doesn't happen often enough to offset the new garments constantly being churned out. Supporting environmentally aware design-ers is a good start to making a change. Our buying choices really matter!

FATAL CONVENIENCE: CHILDREN'S CLOTHING

The first thing to keep in mind whenever we discuss children and Fatal Conveniences is this obvious fact: kids are small. Tiny, you could say.

This means any toxic exposure that might harm us is going to be doubly dangerous to them. They're in the early stages of physical and mental development, so their growing brains, bones, and organs are more vulnerable than ours. Their immune systems aren't yet up to full strength. Their reproductive systems are immature and in greater danger than ours from chemicals known to be hormone disruptors. Their skin is softer and thinner than ours, so it's more likely to absorb whatever rubs up against it.

It's common sense, then: we need to be even more vigilant with our children's clothing than we are with our own. But are we? Not that I can tell.

A landmark study of chemical content in children's clothing was done by the Washington State Department of Ecology. Researchers tested every kind of garment imaginable, from shirts and pants to underwear and socks to pajamas and coats. Here's what they discovered.

- Antimony, the number one toxin on the list, a metal and known carcinogen, showed up in 72 percent of the samples analyzed. It's usually in printed fabrics—in other words, all those cute shirts, socks, and pajamas featuring cartoon characters, unicorns, or puppies. It's also present in clothing treated with flame retardants, common in kiddie pajamas. Today, many large retailers and manufacturers have banned flame retardants because of their antimony content, but not all. Antimony is also found in plastic bibs, which make for easy cleanup but are bad for babies' health.
- The researchers discovered other metals in the clothing, too: lead (which causes brain damage and developmental disorders), as well as cobalt, arsenic, cadmium, mercury, and molybdenum, all of which also pose health hazards.
- One-third of the garments tested contained phthalates, chemicals used to soften plastics. They're in literally thousands of consumer products, everything from cosmetics to vinyl flooring—pretty much anywhere plastic is found. These chemicals have been proven to decrease testosterone production and impair the development of the male reproductive organs, something to keep in mind if you want grandchildren someday.
- Phthalates also affect the development of children's brains, putting them at higher risk for learning, behavioral, and attention disorders. In 2017, the federal government banned the use of phthalates in children's toys and other products, but for some reason not in their clothing. Remember this, too, when you're feeding the little one: phthalates are used in making plastic food containers, and they leach into the food.

A follow-up report to that study, titled "Chemicals Revealed: The State of Chemicals in Children's Products," by Toxic-Free Future, identified more than five thousand widely available products, including not only shoes and clothing but also car seats, bedding, and arts and crafts supplies, that contain one or more of sixty-six "chemicals of high concern to children."

In addition, children's clothing, just like what we adults wear, often contains the "forever chemicals," PFASs, that make our garments waterproof or stain resistant, something that sounds particularly useful for kids. But as I mentioned previously, they're linked to kidney and testicular cancer, liver damage, and a long list of other serious ailments.

How About the Environment?

I'll refrain from sounding the same alarms over and over; basically the environmental issues are the same (except maybe in smaller sizes).

Okay, So What Should We Do?

When possible, buy organic cotton or other natural fiber garments. That includes bibs, despite the fact that a cotton bib is harder to keep clean than one made of plastic. Avoid anything stain resistant, wrinkle free, or waterproof, all of which contain chemicals that are dangerous for humans of all ages. Especially beware of flame-retardant clothes. I know I'm suggesting that you create a lot of work for yourself, but when it comes to keeping your kids and their clothes clean and healthy, it's worth it.

Another good idea is to dress your child in hand-me-downs (as lots of parents do already, since the little tykes outgrow their clothes long before they wear out). At least some of the toxins will already have been washed out.

FATAL CONVENIENCE: COTTON T-SHIRT

It's so soft, friendly, and comfortable, so stylish yet simple and timeless—it's the universal garment, the one thing worn by every human being no matter how old or young, rich or poor, fashionable or clueless. It started out as men's underwear and took off because it's so easy to care for and looks so good. It doesn't matter if we bought it in a three-pack at the drugstore or paid hundreds of dollars for it at some chi-chi boutique. It's maybe the only thing everyone in the world can agree on: we love cotton T-shirts.

Yet behind those lovable garments there's a world of hurt being done: to the environment, to the workers who make them, and even to those of us wearing them. We may love T-shirts, but they sure don't love us back.

The cotton T-shirt is a perfect example of a truth that applies pretty much to every single thing I'm writing about in this book. The personal and the environmental are one and the same: if a thing is harmful to our bodies, it's bad for the environment; if it contaminates the air, the water, the soil, or wildlife, it's contaminating us as well. The story of the T-shirt is a good reminder that we are part of nature, the same as any tree or fish or sea. People discuss "the environment" as though it's something separate from us. But it's not. There's not a bit of difference.

We believe that anything made of cotton must be okay, for the simple reason that it's a natural fiber that comes from a plant. That's true as far as it goes, but most of the time we don't wear it as nature made it.

First, nearly all cotton used in clothing has been sprayed with pesticides, some of which are carcinogenic or cause reproductive problems in humans. In fact, cotton farming is a major guilty party in the worldwide pesticide crisis. In the United States, 97 percent of the crop is grown with the aid of toxic agricultural chemicals. Globally, one-quarter of all pesticides are used on cotton fields.

Second, it takes a huge amount of fresh water to grow enough cotton to make a T-shirt. In some parts of the world drought is always a threat. But of course, cash crops drink first.

Then the cotton has to be processed and dyed. The textiles used in T-shirts are treated with the same toxic chemicals used on all other types of fabric. In total, eight thousand different chemicals are used in various stages of T-shirt production. We wearers have no idea which ones, except we know that the worst of them—PFOAs, phthalates, formaldehyde— are used in pretty much all industrial fabric manufacture.

As I started this chapter by saying, once upon a time all our clothing was dyed using plants, minerals, even insects. Now tinting is strictly synthetic; according to research conducted for the World Bank, seventy-two toxic chemicals are used in fabric dyeing alone. Azo dyes make up between 60 and 80 percent of colorants used today. They are synthetic, nitrogen based, and release chemicals called aromatic amines, which can also be found in pesticides and are carcinogenic. They have been banned in the European Union, Japan, China, Vietnam, and India. These chemicals have been found to cause skin problems, which is no wonder considering how much time they spend rubbing against our skin, our largest organ. They are absorbed as they lie against our skin for prolonged periods.

Perfluorinated chemicals, such as formaldehyde and chlorinated paraffin, are used in the finishing water rinse. They are neurotoxins, endocrine disruptors, carcinogens, and bioaccumulative, meaning that they build up inside our bodies. Chlorine, another toxic chemical, is used for whitening cotton. It can cause breathing problems, even asthma.

The fact that nearly all T-shirts are made in the developing world tells you that workers' safety is not a top priority and working conditions are probably worse—more dangerous, more toxic—than they would be in developed countries. Not only is workers' health disregarded, but the health of the environment is ignored, too.

All those dyes and chemicals used to make our T-shirts? They don't degrade. Instead, they go into the land and into the waterways outside the factories, where they form a toxic film that blocks out light, killing animal and plant life. These chemicals then make their way from the water to the food chain; chemicals from dyes have been found in vegetables and fruits.

None of this is unique to T-shirts, of course. But it's the shirts' popularity that makes them such a threat to human, animal, and plant life. Can you guess how many T-shirts are sold all around the world in just one year? Two billion!

Okay, So What Should We Do?

Stop wearing T-shirts? That'll never happen, but you can make them less of a scourge. You can try to stop buying so many of them. Or you can buy used instead. In many ways, shopping vintage is the best way to attack the problem of waste in fashion; the most sustainable piece is one that doesn't have to be made in the first place.

Even better (and cheaper), you can wear hand-me-downs. Just the other day I went online and bought some upcycled vintage Harley T-shirts. Time has off-gassed all the chemicals. Buying them did two nice things for me: I felt good purchasing a vintage shirt, and it reminded me of my dad because we rode our Harleys together. (And the fact I am writing this book for you is because of him. It's really all connected!)

If you must buy new, wear only organic cotton. Aside from not using pesticides, it requires a lot less water to process than conventional cotton does.

Some companies now take old T-shirts and either repair them, turn them into something else, or recycle the fabric. As you might expect, their products are some of the finest-looking shirts you can find. The fact that they're made by creative people who are trying to protect the planet—which also means protecting you and me—only makes the clothes cooler.

Look for the Global Organic Textile Standard (GOTS) or OEKO-TEX certification on clothing labels, as these organizations prohibit the use of toxic chemicals in the clothing they certify. GOTS takes things a step further by considering the fiber source and other layers of production; it's really the platinum standard for a truly sustainable textile, from the farm to the finished product. Also check out Cradle to Cradle Certified, an initiative that came out of William McDonough and Michael Braungart's now-classic book *Cradle to Cradle: Remaking the Way We Make Things*. It measures material health, as well as social justice, material reuse, renewable energy, and water stewardship.

Look closely at brand websites to understand their chemical policies. Target announced a chemical reduction policy with the goal of full ingredient transparency (including fragrances). It is also removing PFCs and flame retardants across its product lines. Other mission-driven brands active in pursuing safer and more ethical manufacturing practices include Outerknown, Stella McCartney, Patagonia, Mara Hoffman, Eileen Fisher, Prana, and Coyuchi. Fully transparent companies make their fiber and chemical strategies easily available on their websites.

Throughout this book, my advice is limited mostly to things we can do as individuals to protect ourselves from harmful products. But we can also take action on a bigger scale by urging companies to do better. You may think they don't listen, but in fact they do, because they figure that for every person who gets in touch to complain, there are many more who feel the same but never bother to say so.

FATAL CONVENIENCES: BRAS

Bras may not seem exactly like conveniences, and for many women they're just the opposite: inconvenient, uncomfortable, and unwanted but necessary. Or so we've been led to believe. They've been around since sometime in the fourteenth century, starting out as a simple bandeau, a band of fabric worn over the breasts. Obviously, they've come a long way since then, though not necessarily to anyone's benefit, especially not the wearers'.

You have chest muscles that support your breasts, but can you guess what happens when you wear a bra? The muscles no longer have to do their job, and that's not good; nonuse weakens them. That's why some experts say that wearing a bra actually causes breast tissue to sag more than it would if those muscles had been working all along.

The problems go beyond that. The synthetic fabric in your bra may have been treated with formaldehyde, which is carcinogenic and can also cause a rash. The fact that the garment is one that you wear tight against your skin, in a place that's warm and moist, means you are increasing the risk of skin irritation. With the rise of athleisure wear came the popularity of the sports bra, a garment that is, in a way, a no-frills throwback to the original bandeau. But it still contains spandex and other synthetic materials.

The difficulty in finding a bra of the proper size is a common complaint. I recently saw a statistic that 80 percent of women are wearing the wrong size. But the problem goes beyond simple discomfort. Wearing a tight bra all day has actually been associated with an increased risk of developing breast cancer. And there's something called Mondor's disease, an inflammation of the veins in the breast and chest wall, that may be caused by wearing ill-fitting bras.

How About the Environment?

There's nothing inherently worse about bras than everything else in this chapter. The same toxic chemicals found in other apparel are in bras, too, and have the same impact on the health of the planet when they are made of synthetic materials that are thrown away and add to the pollution.

Okay, So What Should We Do?

Start by asking yourself: Do you really need to ever wear a bra? If the answer is yes, make sure you're wearing the right size, meaning one that does the job without hurting you. And try leaving it off for as long as you feel comfortable going without. Your chest muscles will grow stronger, and your breasts will benefit. In what might be the only benefit of covid, many women worked from home instead of the office, at which point bras became pointless, pun totally intended.

Buy bras made with natural fibers only—organic cotton, hemp, or silk—and free of chemicals such as formaldehyde. Padded and push-up bras are probably stuffed with polyester or some other synthetic fabric, so maybe it's time to give those up. Steer clear of underwire bras, especially if you're nursing, because they may impede the milk glands. Since your breasts change over the course of your menstrual cycle, you may need bras in more than one size.

Here's a final bit of advice: If you're not already doing strength training of your upper body muscles, it's time to begin. You'll be healthier overall, and your pecs will do a better job of supporting your breasts.

FATAL CONVENIENCES: DISPOSABLE DIAPERS

Sure, newborns are cute, sweet, and lovable, but they have an extremely inconvenient habit: they pee and poop whenever they feel like, and it's our job to deal with it. This has always been the case, though it wasn't until the 1500s that diapers appeared on the scene. Tell young people today how parents managed back in the age of cloth diapers, and they'll stare at you in shock. *Yuck!*

Only in the early 1960s did we start making use of what seemed like a brilliant solution: disposable diapers. Parents heaved a great sigh of relief. But baby? Probably not.

Disposable diapers have a challenging job: they must fit snugly and stay on an active infant, contain whatever the child unleashes, and then store it securely in a layer of absorbent material a safe distance from baby's skin. Some feature fragrance, moisturizer, even a wetness indicator. To do all that, they require a long list of synthetic materials: adhesives, plastics, polymers, chemicals including phthalates, chlorine, and dyes. There may be some natural fiber in there as well, such as cotton, which indicates the likely presence of pesticides.

Keep in mind that a baby will be wearing one of these things wrapped tightly around his or her most delicate parts twenty-four hours a day for about two years. (The average baby goes through around two thousand diapers annually, fueling a $71-billion-a-year industry.) That's an intense exposure to a mystery mix of who knows what. The federal Consumer Products Safety Commission doesn't require manufacturers to test diapers for safety. There's not even a requirement to list the substances they're made from. So we're on our own.

The authors of a study published in the journal *Reproductive Technology* in 2019 tested four different brands of diapers and detected the volatile organic compounds (VOCs) toluene and xylene, both of which are known reproductive toxicants and can be absorbed through the skin—in all four. As a reminder, VOCs are organic compounds that are released into the air even at room temperature, meaning that we're all unknowingly breathing them in during the course of daily living. According to the researchers, "the physical location of the exposure site, the high absorption rate of the genitalia for chemicals, and the long-term exposure period" are all cause for serious concern.

Because diapers contain phthalates to make the plastic lining softer and more pliable, they can cause dermatitis and rashes. According to one study, two phthalates in particular—DBP and DEHP—were in all brands of diapers tested. Both are classified by California regulators as reproductive and developmental toxicants. A French governmental agency tested disposable diapers and found formaldehyde and the notorious pesticide glyphosate, also known as Roundup, which I mentioned earlier in the book and is maybe the most lethal chemical ever used in agriculture. Both those chemicals are cancer causing.

Glyphosate? In diapers?

A final scary thing about disposable diapers is that they contain hormone disruptors. In the journal *Environmental Science and Technology*, it was reported that the plastics used in disposable diapers were found to be capable of raising levels of estrogen and lowering those of male hormones—not just in the lab but in human subjects. That's not a great start in life for your child.

How About the Environment?

Disposable diapers are the third largest consumer item found in land-fills. They generate sixty times as much solid waste as reusable diapers, require twenty times as many raw materials, including crude oil and wood pulp, and will take five hundred years to decompose. Disposable diapers even contain traces of dioxin, a cancer-causing by-product of the paper-bleaching process. And although human waste goes through sewage treatment systems, diapers go straight into landfills, where at some point the feces they contain will leach into the earth and eventually into our water supply.

Okay, So What Should We Do?

You probably won't want to hear this, but it would be healthier for everyone if you used cloth diapers rather than putting disposable ones made of toxic substances against your baby's delicate flesh. Cloth diapers aren't without their own environmental cost, I understand. Cotton agriculture uses huge amounts of water and pesticides and has a hefty carbon footprint. But a cloth diaper can be reused anywhere between fifty and two hundred times. If you buy diapers made of organic cotton, even better. There's no such thing as a recycled disposable diaper, at least not yet.

If you're not prepared to go that route, here are some suggestions from the Environmental Working Group's guide to safe diapers. Among its recommendations:

+ Read the packaging closely for a list of the diapers' contents, and if there's no such information, don't buy them.
+ Don't use diapers containing dye, fragrance, lotion, or any other extra, unnecessary features.
+ Choose brands that use unbleached pulp or pulp bleached without using chlorine.

✦ Choose brands that specify no use of phthalates, parabens, or bisphenols—all of which are PFAS chemicals—or flame retardants.

EWG verifies safe disposable diaper brands. For more information on those, go to ewg.org.

You should also consider going without baby wipes. They are hugely popular, I realize, but are bad for your child, your sewer system, and the world. Not so long ago, disposable diapers and baby wipes didn't even exist, and somehow we survived.

FATAL CONVENIENCE: SPANDEX

If your clothes stretch and cling in all the right places and make you look shapely, thank spandex. Also known as Lycra, the brand name dreamed up by DuPont back in the 1950s, or elastane, it's a synthetic concoction manufactured in a complicated chemical process. Mostly it's made of polyurethane, which is a cousin of plastic (for me to explain any further, we'd both need an advanced degree in chemistry). Polyurethane is one of the man-made substances found everywhere, from varnish and insulation to upholstery and bedding.

In apparel, it was popular first in girdles and, once those fell out of fashion, in women's swimwear and athleisure wear (which everyone now wears both in and out of the gym and yoga studio). Today, stretchiness is in style in jeans, fine wool, cotton, and other fabrics, all of which contain some portion (usually not more than 20 percent) of spandex. It's listed clearly on labels, so we don't have to guess.

The downside is the same as the upside: garments made with spandex fit so snugly that the skin can't breathe, moisture gets trapped, and heat builds up. That increases the risk of infections and rashes, including ringworm, which isn't as disgusting as it sounds (no worms are involved; the rash resembles rings on your skin) but still is no fun. Spandex also raises the risk of developing yeast infections and other types of inflammation caused by bacteria or fungus. And of course, when your body heat rises in the gym or on the track, more of the chemicals in your clothing are released—right onto your skin.

Is there any scientific proof that spandex actually causes serious ailments? No. However, as I've asked over and over, do you really want to subject your body to hazardous chemicals if you can avoid them?

How About the Environment?

There's no evidence that spandex workers are in any particular danger from their jobs, although studying its health hazards isn't high on any researchers' list of priorities. But keep in mind that every time you wash anything containing spandex, microparticles are shed and enter our waterways and ultimately wildlife and our water supply. Plus, the fact that the material is 100 percent industrial chemicals means that today's cool and flattering yoga pants will someday end up as more toxic trash making the world a nastier place to live. Around 60 percent of the trash in US waterways is composed of nonbiodegradable textile fibers, and spandex garments and fibers are part of that.

Okay, So What Should We Do?

Obviously, just don't wear spandex or anything containing it unless it's completely unavoidable. It's going to be a challenge for women to find natural fiber swimsuits that do the job, I realize. Some health-conscious companies make them in organic cotton or hemp, but even those need a little spandex content or they'd sag and slip right off in the water. Still, they're a better option than most bathing suits, which are made totally of synthetics such as polyester or nylon *plus* spandex—a really bad combo.

For the gym or yoga studio you can certainly find cotton garments containing just a little spandex (5 percent or even less) or none at all. But as a general rule, because your body heat will release some of the toxic chemicals your workout clothes contain, the less stretchy your outfits are, the better.

FATAL CONVENIENCE: DRY CLEANING

Even though it costs more than washing clothes at home, dropping them off at the dry cleaner's and getting them back fresh, pressed, and looking like new is hard to beat. But what we gain in ease we pay for in exposure to dangerous cancer-causing chemicals, both on the clothing itself and in our environment—to the point where the EPA is currently making an effort to abolish the chemicals that nearly all dry cleaners use.

"Dry" is a misnomer, of course, and has been since ancient Romans cleaned stubborn dirt from their togas using ammonia derived from urine. Since then, a variety of petroleum-based fluids, including gasoline, kerosene, and turpentine, has been used, and they did the job well. But once cleaners started using electrical machines, they ran into a problem: the solvents kept catching fire.

Starting in the 1930s, our clothes have been cleaned using the chloride-based chemical tetrachloroethylene or perchloroethylene—PCE or PERC for short. It does the job, but it's nasty stuff; according to various studies, it's a respiratory and skin irritant, liver and kidney toxicant, and reproductive and developmental toxicant. PCE is considered to be a potential carcinogen for workers; the International Agency for Research on Cancer has termed it "probably carcinogenic to humans." Long-term exposure to PCE is especially risky for the brain; it's been associated with impaired memory, confusion, dizziness, headaches, drowsiness, even the development of color blindness.

Here's what's worrisome even for us consumers: a 2011 study at Georgetown University published in *Environmental Toxicology and Chemistry* found that PCE remains on dry-cleaned clothing, especially on wool, polyester, and cotton (though not silk), and that it builds up on garments rather than evaporating over time, which is why some wearers eventually develop contact dermatitis. The research also showed that PCE is "volatilized from these fabrics under ambient room air conditions," meaning that you inhale toxic fumes emanating from your nice clean clothing.

As I've said before, don't be deceived by the fact that the chemical exposure is relatively small. Scientists agree that we still don't know how the human body responds to the various combinations of untested industrial substances we ingest, inhale, and otherwise come into contact with in our daily lives.

There have been attempts to replace PCE with other chemicals, but these have also proven to be toxic. There are two alternative technologies, however, that have been found to be both effective and safe. One uses liquid carbon dioxide in high-pressure machines and with specialized detergents. This gets clothes clean, with no known harm to humans. The other is professional wet cleaning, or PWC, which also uses high-tech machinery, water, and gentle detergents to do the job, with no damage to the health of consumers, workers, or the environment.

The main drawback of both these methods is financial—it's expensive to switch over from the machinery that uses PCE. And the dry-cleaning industry is made up mostly of small operators, who are in no position to spend big bucks on fancy new equipment. Since the EPA began efforts to phase out the use of PCE, several local and state governments have begun subsidizing dry cleaners' efforts to make the switch.

How About the Environment?

There are more than twenty-five thousand dry cleaners in the United States, and nearly all of them use PCE. Workers have been tested with dangerously high levels of the chemical in their blood, and some communities have been contaminated by the chemical. California has committed to phasing out the use of PCE altogether, and the EPA has already ordered that no cleaners located in residential apartment buildings can continue using it. The agency is headed toward banning the chemical altogether—eventually. By then, however, a great deal of damage will have been done. We can't afford to wait on officials to remove PCE and other powerful solvents from our lives.

Okay, So What Should We Do?

Whenever possible, don't buy garments that say "Dry clean only." Often, these will be made from synthetic fabrics, so you're doing two good deeds at once.

Wash fine wool and cashmere knits at home, gently, by hand—remember, before you bought them they were being worn by sheep and goats, who weren't harmed by soap and water. The garments will also last longer if they are not subjected to harsh chemicals, they will smell better, and they will be softer than if you dry-clean them.

After wearing your clothes, let them air out, preferably in sunlight, rather than automatically taking them to be dry-cleaned. If there's a stain, try using a spot remover; it's not necessary to get the whole garment cleaned for every little smudge.

If something absolutely must be dry-cleaned, try to find a place that uses one of the green alternatives, liquid carbon dioxide or professional wet cleaning (PWC). Look online, but keep in mind that such cleaners are not found everywhere yet. Be wary of any other solvent-based methods that claim to be environmentally friendly, because they probably aren't.

Another thing, a side issue: ask your dry cleaner to stop putting your clothes into plastic bags. How good for the planet can they be? And you're not likely to get the clothes dirty on the way home.

FATAL CONVENIENCE: LEATHER

I'm going to be straight with you: there's not really much evidence that leather is harmful to people who wear it. Around 1 percent might suffer from chromium dermatitis because the chemical used in tanning leather rubs off onto their skin. There's not a lot for the rest of us to worry about. After all, leather is a natural fabric. We've been wearing it for thousands of years. When ancient hunters killed, they used every bit of their prey: skin, bone, muscle, organs, tendons, hoofs, and horns, the works. There was a kind of honor expressed in that attitude.

Obviously, it was on a totally different scale than the current global trade in animal hides. Today, the manufacturing and use of leather, which is anything but honorable, do enormous damage in three main ways.

First, there's the terrible impact on the environment from the processes used to turn hides into clothing, upholstery, and so on. Dead skin would rot if left untreated. Once, a vegetable-based tanning method was used, but today chromium is the main chemical preserving leather for consumer wear. Formaldehyde, coal-tar derivatives, and numerous oils, dyes, and finishes, some of them cyanide based, are also employed. All those chemicals, once used, enter our waterways.

Second, working in a leather tannery is an extremely hazardous way to make a living. Once, there were tanneries all over the United States, nasty places to work in or live near due to the toxic chemicals used in the process. Now most leather comes from China and India, so for us the toll on the environment and on workers' health is out of sight and therefore out of mind, sad to say.

Tannery workers suffer from higher-than-normal rates of respiratory problems from inhaling leather dust, as well as other serious disorders caused by inhaling the solvents and other chemicals used in the processing. Today, these workers are mostly in poor Asian countries, and if they were able to find safer work, they no doubt would do so. Instead, they get sick and die so we can have plenty of leather. Even people who live near the plants reportedly have elevated levels of leukemia.

"Tanning is one of the most toxic industries in the world because of the chemicals involved," according to Ecologist, an environmental news website. "Chrome, known for its cancer-causing abilities, is used in huge amounts as are acids, natrium and ammonium salts. A 2005 study showed 69,000 tons of chrome salts are used annually in 1,600 Indian tanneries. But despite the dangers, workers can still be seen labouring without adequate protective gear."

And third, all that is bad enough. But there's something even more sickening.

I'm encouraged to see how many people today are either giving up meat altogether or eating less of it. For some, it's about health. For others, it's because of the huge carbon footprint and other degradations of the planet caused by the livestock industry.

But for many, it's because they can no longer support the torture and slaughter of defenseless animals. I applaud that, but here's what somehow is forgotten: anything made of leather or suede—jackets, pants, shoes, handbags, luggage, your dog's collar, your child's football, all the rest—also requires that animals be held from birth in filthy, disgusting confinement and then killed for profit.

Eating beef, pork, or lamb . . . wearing leather or suede . . . there's no difference. It blows my mind—people who would never think of wearing fur have no problem with leather, even though it's also part of a living creature that we turn into adornment.

The softest leathers come from the youngest animals, such as newborn calves. They are even cut from their mothers' wombs for their skins. In some cases, the hides do not even come from the advertised sources. In China, dogs and cats are killed for their skins, which are then fraudulently sold to us as conventional leather (trade in those animals' hides is illegal in the United States). The poor creatures are sometimes even skinned alive, because it's cheaper than killing them humanely.

That's the Fatal Convenience here—we conveniently forget that if we want to wear leather, animals must first suffer and die.

As someone who loves all animals, I can't imagine why anyone needs to kill a fellow living being just to wear its skin. I am not back in the 1800s living rough on the plains of Minnesota, needing to wear fur to stay alive. I don't need to kill for my clothing, and neither do you.

How About the Environment?

By now, we're all familiar with the toll that animal farming takes on the planet. It's responsible for the deforestation of the Amazon basin, which is contributing to global pollution as well as the habitat loss of millions of species. The damage is done here at home, too. Raising animals for slaughter comes with a huge carbon footprint; it requires agricultural crops (and heavy pesticide use) to feed the animals and leaves behind vast lakes of excrement that befoul the country.

Okay, So What Should We Do?

Stop buying new leather garments and other products. If you really must wear leather, shop at vintage stores. Even better, try one of the several kinds of nonanimal "leather" already in use, with more being developed all the time. I'm talking about fabrics made from used coffee grounds, seashells, pineapple fibers, algae, or mycelium (threads from mushroom roots). They all fall under the heading of "vegan leather," and they look, feel, and wear like the real thing. Years ago, while I was working on a water purification project in an African village, a man showed me a tree with bark that looked and felt exactly like leather. So you see, there are many choices out there—without the cruelty or the pollution.

POSTSCRIPT

We hardly ever think of our fashion habits when we worry about our impact on the environment. I hope you see now that that's a big mistake. There are plenty of steps we can take, even as clothing consumers, to protect our planet and ourselves. Here are two of them.

Number one: Pay attention to what you buy and wear! Just keep reminding yourself that your personal choices really do make a difference.

Number two: Buy fewer clothes.

According to one estimate, the average American purchases more than sixty garments a year, including shoes. More than one a week! I truly dislike shopping for clothes and do it only when absolutely necessary, so there must be someone out there who is buying both his or her share *and* mine. The fact is that right now, the world has more than enough apparel to clothe us all, without a single new item ever being produced.

Ever!

I get it, sometimes we need new things, and many people take great pleasure in clothes shopping and buying. But we can all begin showing a little restraint. Even skipping just a few purchases will make a difference. Next time, before you decide to buy something new, ask yourself if your life will really suffer if you abstain. Chances are the answer will be no. If we all do this occasionally, we'll make an immediate positive change.

We can also start buying vintage, preowned, or used apparel, call it whatever you like. Right now this is a huge and hopeful trend, especially among young people. Once, this was the specialty of Goodwill and Salvation Army stores serving shoppers who needed to be extra careful with their budgets. Today, almost every city and town all over the world has shops devoted to cool vintage clothing and home furnishings. There's also a vast online world of chic and fashionable marketplaces where you can buy and even rent used designer garments. Obviously, buying used clothes cuts down on the environmental damage caused by apparel manufacture, which we've already discussed: the staggering need for water; the pesticides used to grow conventional cotton; the toxic chemicals needed to treat, bleach, and dye textiles; the plastics and petroleum products contained in synthetic fabrics.

This trend is part of the growing awareness of how all our buying habits affect the environment. It's a far more sustainable way of shopping than buying everything brand new. It's a way to do good while indulging your taste for stylish looks. Meanwhile, "fast fashion," ultracheap clothing meant to be worn for a little while, then discarded, is falling *out* of fashion. That's a very good sign. In fact, it's being replaced by something called "slow fashion," a movement where high style meets environmental awareness.

Or rent your wardrobe; the pioneer at this, Rent the Runway, is now a billion-dollar business, and there are others, too.

When you absolutely must buy new clothing, there's a long list of manufacturers who specialize in environmentally sensitive goods, made responsibly and in ways that also treat textile workers ethically. Garments of natural materials and nontoxic manufacturing processes are some of the coolest-looking clothes on the planet. It's worth the extra effort to find them.

8

HOUSEHOLD PRODUCTS

HOME IS SUPPOSED TO BE THE safest place in the world, where we go to feel secure, protected, and at ease. So how did it end up so dangerous? Maybe that's slightly exaggerated. But home sweet home is definitely not as safe as we imagine.

First, it may be a little *too* comfortable. It contains so many wonderful things, and we love them all so well that we find no reason to leave. Our ancestors were just the opposite, spending most of their time working outdoors and coming in only to eat and sleep.

I'm not suggesting that we go back in time, but the truth is that our biology is not made for this lifestyle. I just read a worrisome statistic: Americans and most other people today spend nearly 92 percent of our time indoors. That probably means we're not getting enough fresh air and sunlight to keep us healthy. And we're not being as physically active as we should be.

Once, home was a shelter from the harsh elements. It was a box. Now it's heaven on Earth. It's *too convenient.* Even something as basic as going out to dinner and a movie has been replaced by Uber Eats and HBO in your pajamas.

But the hazards of home go way beyond that. We live in well-built, completely insulated containers filled with furniture and furnishings made using chemicals that have been proven to be harmful to our health.

We keep our houses clean and germ free with products made from toxic chemicals capable of causing everything from rashes to kidney disease.

Your sofa? Phthalates. Your bedsheets? Formaldehyde. Your Tupperware containers? Your laundry detergent? Bad stuff at every turn. Even air fresheners find a way to make your air less safe than when it smelled like plain old air. All those ultrapowerful all-purpose cleaning products that promise to kill germs and mold? What else do you think they might be killing?

Let's find out.

FATAL CONVENIENCES: HOME CLEANING PRODUCTS

Clean is good. How about *too* clean? What happens if the ways we reach maximum cleanliness wind up scouring us, too?

As we saw in the chapter on personal care products, we tend to go overboard when it comes to ridding our bodies of grit and grime. It's no surprise that we do the same when it comes to our surroundings. Is it because we're germophobic? Or maybe it's peer pressure thanks to all those big corporate marketing budgets.

Either way, the supermarket shelves are full of products that eradicate dirt, leaving our world sparkling and spotless. But how do they go about it?

Of the substances regulated by the federal Toxic Substances Control Act, there were at last count 86,228 different chemicals listed. Can you imagine trying to monitor all of them? About half are currently being produced and included in products we use—still a huge number. Of those, almost eight thousand have what the government calls "confidential identities," meaning that the manufacturer doesn't have to tell anybody the precise makeup of the toxic substance because it's considered a trade secret.

Under that law, it's the job of the EPA to assess the risks to our health and our environment caused by substances found in consumer products.

But don't feel too reassured; the EPA has reviewed only a small percentage of those chemicals and forced even fewer off the market.

In other words, nobody is protecting you from cleaning products that do more harm than good. If the chemicals in them are capable of wiping out every bit of crud found in the average home, imagine what they can do to you—your skin, your lungs, your eyes—and how they might affect your kids and your pets, too.

The main danger is the presence of volatile organic compounds, or VOCs. These are man-made chemicals often found not only in home cleaning products but also in paint, dry-cleaning fluid, and a long list of other hazardous things we encounter every day. Their volatility means that they off-gas, or spew as invisible vapor, their contents into the air we breathe—straight into our lungs.

According to an article in the journal *Occupational & Environmental Medicine*, the VOCs and other chemicals released when we use cleaning supplies contribute to chronic respiratory problems, allergic reactions, headaches, and more. Preservatives containing formaldehyde are also commonly added to multiuse cleaning products.

The Environmental Working Group does a great job of testing household cleaning products. An evaluation of twenty-one of them found that they emitted more than 450 chemicals into the air, including compounds linked to asthma, developmental and reproductive damage, even cancer. Studies have shown that infants exposed in the womb to cleaning products used by their mothers may suffer from lowered birth weight, lowered IQ, and respiratory symptoms that may persist throughout childhood.

Are you starting to catch my drift? One product, many untested chemicals; many products, endless exposures to chemicals, many of which are known to be harmful.

Cleaning supplies and household products containing VOCs and other toxic substances include just about everything you use to keep your house gleaming. And that's not all they contain. Here's a rundown of just some of the toxicity we welcome into our homes.

All-purpose cleaners, the ones meant for every surface, commonly include ammonia, ethylene glycol monobutyl ether acetate, sodium hypochlorite, and trisodium phosphate. They're sometimes listed on the labels. None of these is safe for us to be around. None!

Ammonia is found in lots of home cleaning products; just the smell tells us that serious cleaning is going on. But in reality, it's a heavy-duty industrial-strength chemical that can pose serious dangers. According to the CDC, "High levels of ammonia can irritate and burn the skin, mouth, throat, lungs, and eyes. Very high levels of ammonia can damage the lungs or cause death. . . . The level of exposure depends upon dose, duration, and work being done."

As with many cleaning products, the biggest danger is to people who use the chemicals in the workplace, hour after hour and year after year. But even smaller doses threaten our health unless we're careful.

Rug- and upholstery-cleaning products can contain tetrachloroethylene or perchloroethylene, also known as PEC or PERC, which is also the main chemical used in dry cleaning. According to the CDC, exposure may cause irritation to the eyes, skin, nose, throat, and respiratory system. Naphthalene and ammonium hydroxide are also found in these products. The EPA classifies naphthalene as a possible human carcinogen. Merely inhaling the fumes from these products may cause dizziness, nausea, loss of appetite, and disorientation. Though you might be tempted to say, "Big deal, those all wear off," you must wonder what else in your brain is being affected by these chemicals. There's also evidence that links them to liver damage and cancer.

Bleach, the kind used for laundry but also in general cleaning products, contains the chemical sodium hypochlorite in various concentrations, ranging from 0.7 percent to 5.25 percent. The potential for damage to our health rises along with the percentage, which is usually noted on the label. Chlorine bleach liquid and the vapors it creates can irritate the eyes, skin, and throat, which will come as no surprise to anyone who uses it.

When bleach is mixed with ammonia, toxic gases called chloramines are produced and cause symptoms such as:

+ Coughing
+ Nausea
+ Shortness of breath
+ Chest pain
+ Wheezing
+ Even pneumonia and fluid in the lungs!

When bleach is mixed with acids, as in some drain and toilet cleaners, the chlorine is off-gassed. Even at low levels and for short periods of time, it will irritate the mucous membranes—meaning your eyes, throat, and nose—and cause coughing, breathing problems, burning and watery eyes, and runny nose. High levels of exposure can cause chest pain, severe breathing difficulties, and vomiting. *Very* high levels can even cause death.

The main ingredient in automatic and hand dishwashing detergents is phosphate. Automatic dishwashing detergents have been known to cause skin irritations or burns; dish detergents for washing by hand are milder.

Furniture cleaners may contain petroleum distillates, which can irritate your mucous membranes when inhaled and may be absorbed through the skin. These chemicals can also affect the nervous system, causing headache, dizziness, nausea, and loss of balance and coordination. They may even affect the liver and kidneys.

Furniture polish (not cleaner) typically contains one or more of the following: ammonia, naphtha, nitrobenzene, petroleum distillates, and phenol. Naphtha may contain benzene, a carcinogen. Repeated exposure may damage the nervous system and affect the kidneys.

Toilet cleaners may contain sodium hypochlorite, hydrochloric acid, or bleach, all of which can be irritating to eyes, skin, and throat.

Chlorine and alkyl ammonium chlorides are the common fungicide chemicals found in mold and mildew removers, which can cause breathing problems.

Clogged-drain cleaners contain lye and sulfuric acid, both of which are heavy duty. Lye burns; that's why it's effective, but also why it's so dangerous. Sulfuric acid not only irritates skin and eyes but can also damage the kidneys, liver, and digestive tract. These chemicals produce fumes that can burn skin and can cause blindness if they accidentally get into your eyes. Of course, you would never use this stuff so carelessly. Still, do you want something so powerful in your house if it's unnecessary?

Window and glass cleaners usually contain ammonia and isopropanol, a form of alcohol, which are irritating to the eyes, skin, nose, and throat.

All-purpose cleaners and disinfecting wipes contain asthmagens, chemicals that can worsen asthma and even cause it. Studies show that using traditional cleaning sprays just once a week may increase your risk of developing adult-onset asthma. Common asthmagens and respiratory irritants in cleaning products include quaternary ammonium compounds, also called quats, ethanolamines, glutaral, and sodium hypochlorite (chlorine bleach).

Toilet cleaners, oven cleaners, and heavy-duty degreasers containing hydrochloric acid, phosphoric acid, sodium or potassium hydroxide, or ethanolamines can all cause lung irritation.

How About the Environment?

I've just listed the harsh and toxic chemicals our cleaning products include. What kind of impact do you imagine they have once they go down our drains and into the world? Many of the products we use, such as laundry and dishwasher detergents, contain phosphorus or nitrogen, which can harm aquatic life. Surfactants, commonly found in cleaning products, biodegrade slowly and cause similar damage; one such chemical, alkylphenol ethoxylates, is even an endocrine disruptor. When wastewater is properly treated, these chemicals are usually removed, but that's not always the case.

Okay, So What Should We Do?

Start with this thought: If opening a container of a cleaning product immediately makes your eyes water or your nose burn, or gives you the sensation of being in the presence of something superpotent, pay attention! If it seems toxic, it probably is. At that point, ask yourself if your house is really filthy enough to require such high-powered cleaning. The answer is likely a definite *no*.

Instead, use warm, soapy water and see how that works. I'm betting that it will do most jobs just as well as the toxic household staples do. If that's not enough, baking soda and water is a great abrasive scrubber. A solution of white vinegar and water mixed in a spray bottle does as good a job on glass as any industrial-strength cleaner. It's also good for bathroom surfaces such as porcelain and tile. And it's cheap. If you want your cleaning product to smell nice, add a few drops of essential oil, such as lavender or tea tree oil, to the spray bottle. And believe it or not, straight vodka is a great cleaning fluid.

If you need something stronger, stick with the old-school cleansers such as Bon Ami, which contains natural materials such as ground feldspar and baking soda, with no unnecessary ingredients.

If you still want to use commercial products, read the labels. There, amid all the multisyllable chemical names, you will probably find a few of those I've been trying to warn you against. Look instead for products that have either no or reduced VOCs, irritants, flammables, or fragrances. Today, there are forward-thinking companies that put this information onto their labels.

Be especially wary of antibacterial products containing triclosan. They're the reason we're all in danger from drug-resistant bugs. Triclosan has even been linked to increased allergen sensitivity and disruption of the thyroid function. If you use plain soap and water, the bacteria in your home won't harm you.

Don't use products that contain quaternary ammonium compounds, or quats. These chemicals are associated with asthma, as well as reduced fertility and birth defects in animals.

If you do use a noxious commercial product, keep the area well ventilated with an open window or two and maybe a fan. And wear rubber gloves while using it.

Instead of using one of those insanely powerful (and toxic) drain cleaners to clear a clog, try an old-school mechanical snake, which you can buy in any hardware store. If that's not working, pour a cup of baking soda and then a cup of white vinegar down the drain, then plug it for half an hour. Once the bubbles die down, run the hot water.

Finally, check out the Environmental Protection Agency's list of products that meet its Safer Choice requirements for cleaning and other needs at epa.gov/saferchoice.

FATAL CONVENIENCE: CARPETING

You know that great new-carpet smell? It means your rugs are off-gassing toxic chemicals into your nasal passages and lungs and those of your loved ones, pets included. You're inhaling PFAS "forever chemicals" linked to cancer, developmental disorders, and endocrine disruption. You're taking in formaldehyde, too, as well as phthalates. All so stains won't stick, meaning that your rug will be more pristine than you are.

In 2021, the California Department of Toxic Substances Control adopted new regulations on carpets and rugs containing PFASs "due to concerns about the hazard traits of PFASs and their widespread presence in the environment, humans, and other living organisms. Carpets and rugs treated with PFASs for stain- or soil-resistance are potential long-term sources of widespread human and ecological exposures to this class of chemicals." California tends to be the pioneer of protecting consumers from harmful chemicals in everyday products, so no matter where we live, we can take this tip and be careful when it comes to rugs as well as the padding and adhesives that go beneath them.

How About the Environment?

One source states that more than 4 billion pounds of carpeting are discarded annually in the United States, and of that, less than 5 percent is recycled. Where do the rest of our used rugs wind up? Either in landfills or burned in incinerators—meaning that all those toxic chemicals that once filled our homes with off-gassing now fill our air and land and probably, at some point, our water, too.

Okay, So What Should We Do?

First, ease up on the carpeting. Use flooring made of natural materials such as bamboo, wood, tile, natural linoleum, even cement, leaving as much of it uncovered as possible. That means using area rugs instead of wall-to-wall, of course, and rugs should be made of wool, sisal, jute, cotton, or some other nonsynthetic fiber. Use felt or wool padding instead of polyester, or choose carpets with a natural rubber backing.

Don't buy rugs that have been treated with stain-resistant chemicals—you'll be inhaling the VOCs for a long time. Instead, either wipe your feet well before entering your home or leave your shoes at your home's entrance and keep your rugs clean that way. Otherwise, all the dirt, dust, pollen, and other junk that gets caught in your carpet will become a permanent part of your environment.

Once you've invested in natural fiber carpets and take precautions to keep them clean and in good condition, they'll last longer than synthetics since they are more durable—which is good because they're going to cost you more money—but they're worth it.

FATAL CONVENIENCE: AIR-CONDITIONING

Considering that intense heat waves can kill people, it's hard to knock air-conditioning as a Fatal Convenience. It's probably kept more people alive than it's harmed. But that doesn't mean it's without its downsides. On the one hand, when it's blazing hot and crazy humid outside, who doesn't turn on the AC? As the planet heats up, we'll need it more than ever. Depending on where you live, it may run nonstop from May through September—nearly half the year. On the other hand, you're completely altering the air inside your home, meaning the air inside your lungs, too—and often, you're making it worse.

Air-conditioning doesn't just cool the air, it dehumidifies it, too. In fact, that was its first purpose, back in 1902, when an engineer named Willis Carrier designed an apparatus to keep paper from shrinking in the summer. His invention worked because when hot, humid air hit chilled coils, the humidity was stripped away. Carrier went on to cofound the first air-conditioner company, which still dominates the industry.

It wasn't until the 1940s that air conditioners became small and cheap enough to be used in homes, and today virtually every American house has at least one, or a central AC system. As poverty rates fall elsewhere in the world, they're catching on everywhere, especially in parts of the southern hemisphere, where it gets *really* hot.

The main health perils of air conditioners have to do with how well they are maintained. If filters are regularly cleaned and replaced when necessary, there's not much harm done. Often, however, upkeep is neglected. When that happens, all the dirt, dust, and allergens that go from the outside atmosphere into the system come spewing out at you.

If you spend any amount of time in an office, a school, or some other public place where you have no control over the AC, you're at the mercy of somebody who may not be as concerned about your health as you are. A 2014 study found that women working in offices with central air-conditioning had higher-than-average rates of absence due to sickness and more visits to ear, nose, and throat doctors. In another study, 8 percent of people who worked in air-conditioned environments suffered from daily headaches.

The likely reason is that air-conditioning's power to dehumidify dries out the mucus membranes in our noses, throats, and ears. When that happens, we lose some of our ability to fight off infections. It also leads to headaches and lethargy.

There's even a phenomenon known as *sick building syndrome*, where our totally sealed and controlled indoor environments become hotbeds of health problems. Thanks to AC, most buildings today are sealed off from the outside world, which does us no good.

Beyond all that, spending so much time in cool environments lowers our natural tolerance for heat, meaning that once we're hooked on air-conditioning, it becomes progressively harder to give it up. Our internal thermostat becomes desensitized from lack of use, and we produce less sweat.

How About the Environment?

Early air conditioners used Freon, a chlorofluorocarbon that depletes the ozone layer and thereby increases global warming. In the 1980s, the infamous "ozone hole" over Antarctica was detected, leading to a worldwide ban on Freon. Its replacement, hydrofluorocarbons (HFCs), don't deplete the ozone, but they do absorb the sun's radiation and keep heat from escaping from our atmosphere—which only leads to increased demand for air-conditioning. The EPA has begun requiring manufacturers to phase out HFCs and replace them with other alternatives.

Then there is the extraordinary energy requirement created by our desire for totally controlled, seriously cool air even during the hottest months. Once upon a time, we took sweating during the summer for granted. We all did it, so nobody felt singled out. And sweating is good for our health because it helps rid our bodies of toxins and waste.

Air-conditioning in the United States uses as much energy as that in the entire continent of Africa, and the International Energy Agency projects that before long, global air-conditioning will use about 13 percent of all electricity worldwide. As the nations of the southern hemisphere come out of poverty, their citizens will begin buying air conditioners to escape the ever-increasing heat. And who can blame them?

Today, perspiration is optional. Unless you are required to be outdoors in summer, it's possible to go from home to car to office or store or wherever else it is you're going in constant air-conditioned comfort—and never be exposed to hot weather for more than a few seconds at a time. Personally, I love to sweat. It means that I'm alive and my body is functioning.

Okay, So What Should We Do?

How about this: Don't turn on the AC! Or leave it off until it's truly painful living without it. First see if opening a few windows and turning on a fan or two is enough to make life tolerable. Try wearing less clothing, especially at home.

Investing in the most efficient AC systems could cut our future demand in half. And more energy-efficient windows and proper shades can be massively helpful, especially in the summer.

Here are some tips from the US Department of Energy.

+ Install window coverings such as shades or blinds to prevent heat gain through your windows during the day.
+ Keep your house warmer than normal when you are away and lower the thermostat setting only when you return home. A programmable thermostat allows you to do this automatically and without sacrificing comfort.
+ Vacuum your air intake vents regularly to remove dust buildup. Ensure that furniture and other objects are not blocking the airflow through your air conditioners or central air-conditioning registers.
+ Seal cracks and openings around windows and doors to prevent warm air from leaking into your home. Add caulk or weather stripping to seal air leaks.

+ Maintain and clean air filters annually; this is important for energy efficiency and to keep possible allergens at bay.
+ Look into buying a lower-emissions system with a refrigerant packed in factory-sealed, leakproof tubing.
+ When it's time to replace an old air conditioner, hire a professional to remove the coolant safely so that none of it leaks into the environment.

FATAL CONVENIENCE: LAUNDRY DETERGENT

We've all seen old photos of women on riverbanks doing laundry by soaking it in the river and beating it on rocks. Looks like fun for maybe the first five minutes but after that, total arm-busting drudgery. Compare it to today, when we can just toss our dirty clothes into a machine, add detergent, hit a button or two, and like magic—clean clothing, ready to dry in yet another machine and then wear. It's hard to begrudge ourselves a little convenience, especially when laundry day comes around. How many of us live near a river anyway?

The machines are fine, I guess. The detergents are not.

We've been washing clothes for as long as we've been wearing them, though we haven't always been as fastidious as we are today. We used to make all our soaps at home of animal fats and ash from wood fires, which contained a cleaning agent, potassium carbonate. Sounds like a lot of work, but at least the ingredients were natural.

The first detergent using industrial chemicals was made by Germans during World War I, because they needed to save animal fats for more pressing needs. It was called Nekal and was only a so-so cleaning product but was an effective wetting agent that is still used in industry today.

After the war, the US consumer product giant Procter & Gamble brought that detergent home, re-created it in its labs here, and introduced the first American-made laundry soap, Dreft, a powder. Before long, the company added sodium tripolyphosphate to the detergent and called it Tide. The detergent captured 30 percent of the US laundry soap market and remains the best seller here today.

As usually happens, once a necessity becomes a big consumer product category, health hazards begin creeping in. In 2008, researchers at the University of Washington released a study revealing that the top-selling laundry products emit dozens—*dozens*—of different chemicals that can damage our health. Of the 1,147 laundry products evaluated in the Environmental Working Group's guide to healthy cleaning, only 185 earned an A rating, meaning that the rest had low or no concern for ingredients that may cause cancer, developmental and reproductive difficulties, respiratory problems, skin irritation and allergies, and environmental hazards.

That should give you a good idea of what you're up against in the laundry aisle. Our clothes come out clean, fresh, and smelling sweet—and full of chemicals capable of causing everything from a rash to cancer.

Companies tend to use sodium laureth sulfate (SLES) in detergents because it's a cheap way to create foam, which we all take as a sign of hardcore cleansing action. The main problem is that when it goes through the process called ethoxylation, there's a potential for contamination with a possible carcinogen called 1,4-dioxane.

Detergents may also contain optical brighteners, which sound like a contradiction in terms, colorless dyes derived from the chemical stilbene, which can cause irritation of the respiratory tract, skin, and eyes. These additives absorb ultraviolet light and reemit it as visible fluorescence, making our clothes look whiter.

Detergent allergies can arise from surfactants, preservatives such as parabens (you might remember them from the earlier chapter about personal products), which are also endocrine disrupters, and fragrance, which—as I've said over and over—is a sign that potentially harmful chemicals have been included for no practical reason. We need to get over our slavery to smell. The EPA's guide to detergent lists around fifty brands that don't add fragrances. So detergents that still use it should be easy to skip.

How About the Environment?

Once, detergents for laundry and dishwashers contained phosphates, which made water softer and got our clothes cleaner. But once those chemicals reached our waterways, they caused unnatural algae blooms, which in turn starved aquatic life of oxygen. Phosphates have been banned by governments, but the problem remains because other chemicals used in detergents create the same effect. As a result, the algae decompose and create underwater "dead zones" that kill fish and plants. Pretty much every chemical contained in big-brand detergents winds up in our waterways, and they all contribute to the harm.

And of course, liquid detergent tends to come in big plastic jugs, meaning that we defile our surroundings with more pointless pollution when we throw the containers away. Some manufacturers—though not enough of them—now sell the stuff in biodegradable pouches. If we customers demand it, though, maybe that will change.

Okay, So What Should We Do?

When you go shopping, compare labels and find the products that use the fewest ingredients. Some detergents use only three, such as baking soda (sodium bicarbonate), washing soda (sodium carbonate), and soap or vegetable oils. Castile soap and borax are also safe. Avoid any product containing:

+ Phosphates
+ Fragrances
+ Optical brighteners
+ 2-butoxyethanol
+ Diethanolamine

Choose fragrance-free products. If you want clothes that smell like something other than clothes, add a few drops of essential oil, such as lavender, to wool dryer balls.

Use as little detergent as possible, which is probably less than the manufacturer recommends. Unless you work on an oil rig or somewhere else that leaves your garments deeply filthy, try cutting back on detergent and see how your clothes come out.

Even better, hang them outdoors in sunlight and fresh air and see if maybe they'd be acceptable to wear in polite company. If there's a small stain, see if a stain remover stick can do the job.

Buy sustainably produced and packaged detergents that are third party certified by UL Solutions' ECOLOGO or by Green Seal.

To make life really convenient, check out either the EPA's Safer Choice database (epa.gov/saferchoice) or the EWG guide to cleaners (ewg.org/guides/cleaners) to find detergents and other products that perform well and are safe for our health and the environment. Also, see chapter 10 for some of my suggestions.

FATAL CONVENIENCES: DRYER SHEETS

Seriously, how harmful can a flimsy little slip of fabric be? Especially when you consider how soft and sweet smelling it leaves your clothes. Think again, my friend—there's a lot of badness contained in that tiny bit of laundry magic.

Why is it that the most trivial Fatal Conveniences start life in the minds of serious inventors? You'd think they'd have more serious things to think about. In the 1960s, a man named Conrad Gaiser wanted to make things a little easier for his wife by sparing her a trip down four flights of stairs to add liquid softener to the washer on the ground floor of their apartment building at the exact moment the wash cycle ended. He poured some softener onto a piece of cotton fabric, so now she could drop a sheet into the dryer at her leisure. He named his invention Tumble Puffs, patented it, and sold it to Procter & Gamble, which called it the Bounce dryer sheet. The rest is Fatal Convenience history.

Dryer sheets work in kind of a weird way: they are made of woven polyester fabric coated with a chemical that melts in the heat of your dryer and transfers onto your clothes. This gives your garments a slippery surface that feels to us like softness, while also perfuming them and cutting down on static electricity. It's an improvement, I guess, at least superficially.

What's the downside? Start with quaternary ammonium compounds, or quats, which make clothes feel soft and cuddly right out of the washer but can also trigger an asthma attack and may even be harmful to the reproductive system. Check labels for these ingredients and avoid them: distearyldimonium chloride and anything else ending in "-monium chloride." Softeners may also include chemicals such as methylisothiazolinone (it even sounds lethal!) and glutaral, both of which can trigger asthma attacks and allergies. Also steer clear of ingredients described as "biodegradable fabric softening agent" or "cationic surfactant."

Aside from softening, the whole point of dryer sheets is that they make clothing smell fresher and cleaner—which we weirdly require even though we just took them out of the washer. As everywhere else in the world of Fatal Convenience, fragrance usually means trouble. Fabric softeners (whether liquid or sheets) may contain phthalates, which disperse the scent, and galaxolide, a synthetic musk that accumulates in the body. But remember that all fragrance is risky because manufacturers refuse to tell us which chemicals they're using. That's a good reason to skip softeners totally.

How About the Environment?

Softener sheets do their damage to the planet in two ways. First, research by Dr. Anne Steinemann at the University of California, Los Angeles, has shown that more than twenty-five volatile organic compounds are emitted from dryer vents, including nine classified as toxic or hazardous, with the highest concentrations being acetone, acetaldehyde, ethanol, methanol, and limonene. Fragranced laundry products can also emit VOCs including alpha-pinene, linalool, and D-limonene. And terpenes in the sheets can react with ozone to generate pollutants such as formaldehyde and ultrafine particles.

The second way is due to all the single-use polyester sheets that we're adding to every other bit of nonbiodegradable junk we discard. It never ends.

Okay, So What Should We Do?

As I find myself beginning so many of these "Okay, So What Should We Do?" entries, here's my best advice: Stop using dryer sheets! By now it's possible that you've become addicted to the aroma of artificially scented laundry. Go cold turkey for a couple of days, and see if you can kick the habit altogether. Remember, they aren't really making your clothes soft, just slippery.

Try adding a half cup of distilled white vinegar to the washer during the rinse cycle and see if that doesn't make your clothes feel softer.

Use wool dryer balls, which soften clothes and reduce static without using chemicals except for the wool's natural lanolin. Make sure they're unscented, though, or you'll wind up with the same fake fragrance used in the sheets.

FATAL CONVENIENCE: FURNITURE

You sit on it, lie on it, sleep on it, and what would Netflix (watching my amazing series, *Down to Earth*, hopefully) and chill be without it? Its sole purpose is to make you feel so comfortable you never want to move. Does the fact that it may be emitting toxic fumes and carcinogenic dust all over you make a difference?

Once, furniture was made in traditional ways with old-fashioned materials: solid wooden frames held together with nails, screws, and glue; cushions filled with down or natural fibers and covered with cotton, horsehair, velvet, canvas, or wool. It was solid as hell and built to last. People once bequeathed their furniture to their descendants. At some point all that began to change, with furniture being manufactured with synthetic petroleum-based fibers, plastics, and composite "wood," all treated with chemicals never before found in our homes. Manufacturing processes changed, prices came down, but so did safety.

One of the biggest problems with furniture came with an attempt to make it safer: the nearly universal use of flame-retardant fabric treatments. It sounded like such a great idea that California actually required its use, and so, to make life simpler, manufacturers began using it on all their sofas and chairs to be sold anywhere in the country. It was also widely used in other products, including mattresses.

As happens so often with added "benefits," it didn't go exactly as planned. The chemical group is called *chlorinated alkyl phosphates*; these include tris(1,3-dichloro-2-propyl)phosphate, or TDCIPP, and other similar substances. They can be carcinogenic. They can disrupt the endocrine system. And they have been found to damage nerve cells and nervous systems. Some blood tests have showed scary levels of the chemicals, particularly in kids, possibly due to the fact that they often play either on living room furniture or on the floor nearby, where dust settles. All that came about so we could protect people who might fall asleep on a sofa while smoking. It was a nice goal, no doubt, but one that came at a steep price.

Finally, California wised up and decided to end the requirement that furniture be treated with flame retardants. Can you guess what happened next? The companies that made and sold those chemicals sued the state, claiming to be looking out for the safety of consumers, who might otherwise burn up in fires. Once again, industry showed its true colors even in the face of clear danger to the rest of us. The ultimate irony is that the chemicals weren't really much good at fighting the spread of flames. Today, many furniture makers have curtailed their use of flame retardants—but not all.

Most furniture today is made with polyurethane foam padding instead of natural materials. Polyfoam is lightweight, durable, flexible, and supportive. It's also cheap. These are all positives, you could argue. But polyfoam is made from petroleum, which should immediately set off alarms. It's also made using toluene diisocyanate (TDI), which the US National Toxicology Program has classified as "reasonably to be anticipated as a human carcinogen." If that's not bad enough, polyfoam is what is treated with the flame-retardant chemicals.

Manufactured wood products, meaning particleboard and other types of "formed" wood, are treated with formaldehyde. This is considered to be cancer causing for people who work with the chemical and are exposed to higher levels than we find in our homes. But again, we're not just breathing in one particular gas; we're under attack by many other carcinogenic chemicals, too. So why subject ourselves to one more?

Finally, the "forever chemicals" that make fabric stain resistant also make upholstery hazardous to our health. I've already discussed these chemicals, since they're contained in clothing, cosmetics, and other consumer goods. They're yet another convenience that's anything but.

How About the Environment?

Considering that polyfoam and synthetic fabrics are nonbiodegradable, the disposable furniture we buy today will languish in landfills, where it will outlive us by several centuries. I've already discussed what happens when all those chemicals and petroleum-based products are discarded, so no there's need to cover it again. It's grim.

Okay, So What Should We Do?

The current system of blindly buying furniture and everything else in our homes—no matter how toxic they are—must change. That will happen only when we demand better products. Meanwhile, buy used/vintage furniture, preferably made in the old-school way from natural materials. Even if you're buying new furniture, the same rules apply. I realize that it may be more expensive than things made from the hazardous materials

I've discussed. But chances are that it will last a lot longer and without the possibility of making you and your family sick.

When upholstery gets worn out, reupholster the piece. If a wood frame begins to break down, take the furniture to a furniture restorer. They still exist, believe it or not, throwbacks to the days when people had things such as appliances and shoes repaired. That was possible only for well-made possessions, of course, but that way you could use your sofa or easy chair (or shoes!) for decades instead of a couple of years.

If that doesn't work for you, seek out furniture made with solid wood rather than composites or plywood. Look for Forest Stewardship Council (FSC) certification, proof that it came from responsibly managed forests. If that's impossible, look for furniture with lower formaldehyde gas emission labels such as "exterior grade" pressed wood, California Air Resources Board (CARB) Phase 2 Compliant, ultra-low-emitting formaldehyde (ULEF), or no added formaldehyde (NAF).

Air out new furniture if you think it was made using formaldehyde, preferably outdoors or in a well-ventilated area. You can even ask the manufacturer to leave the furniture unsealed in the warehouse for a few days before it's delivered to your home.

You can apply latex-based paint or formaldehyde-free varnish to formaldehyde-containing furniture to create a surface barrier.

Thanks to new fire safety standards in California, many furniture manufacturers across the country now produce sofas and other upholstered furniture without flame-retardant chemicals. Read the label carefully. If you must smoke, do so carefully.

And instead of needing stain-resistant upholstery, try being careful with your furniture. Don't let the kids eat on your sofa, and maybe you shouldn't be eating there, either. If that's not possible, buy furniture with upholstery you can wash.

FATAL CONVENIENCE: NONSTICK COOKWARE

It was one of those labor-saving modern household miracles back in the 1960s: a new product that would make cooking and cleanup easier than homemakers dreamed possible. What could go wrong? Teflon became such a large part of American life that soon it was an adjective, used to describe someone who could slide through shady moments without any bad stuff sticking. Ronald Reagan was called "the Teflon president." A gangster who evaded prison (for a while) was known as a "Teflon Don."

In 1938, a scientist working for DuPont was trying to develop a refrigerant gas. Instead, a happy accident in the lab produced a white powder with no apparent benefits except that it was slippery. A large number of industrial applications were soon found, but it wasn't until 1954 that a French engineer's wife suggested that he try to bond the chemical, called polytetrafluoroethylene (PTFE), to cooking surfaces. Voilà! nonstick pans were born. In 1960, the FDA approved the use of the chemical for food-related purposes, and Teflon took off.

It was a nice little story—until somebody realized that those pans also contained PFOA, one of the "forever chemicals," and that if it got into the food, it was probably exposing people to a long list of health hazards, cancer among them. Now, if those pans were never scratched, they might have been safe, but that's not how things work in the real world. Every little chip or ding of the cooking surface pretty much guaranteed that you'd be eating nonstick chemicals along with your dinner, without ever knowing.

So since 2015, PFOAs in cookware have been replaced by other chemicals from the same family, ones that have not been proven to be dangerous. Of course, that doesn't necessarily mean they're safe. Some nonstick pans now advertise themselves as PFOA free, but PFOA and PTFE are just two of the thousands of polyfluoroalkyl substances used in consumer products, and manufacturers don't have to disclose their use because it is considered to be a trade secret.

There's a manufacturing technique called GenX that claims to make nonstick chemicals safely, without PFOAs. But the EPA's assessment shows that even small doses of GenX chemicals could present serious health risks, including harm to prenatal development, as well as the immune system, liver, kidneys, and thyroid.

So we come back around to the same questions that hang over the rest of this book: Is the convenience worth the cost? Is the reward worth the risk? By now you know my answer: no way! People cooked their food—*safely*—long before Teflon came along.

How About the Environment?

As I've stated more than once, the PFAS chemicals found in Teflon pollute water and don't break down easily—in fact, they're termed *persistent*, meaning that they remain in the environment (and us) for decades. Nearly every American tested has them in his or her blood. They didn't necessarily absorb it from nonstick cookware. It's in so many consumer products that it could have come from anywhere, including tap water.

Okay, So What Should We Do?

To be safest, don't use nonstick surface cookware. There are great alternatives. Ceramic nonstick pots and pans are coated with silica manufactured using a process that creates a nontoxic nonstick surface. The only downside is that the coating lasts only one to three years before losing its slipperiness. Cast-iron pans are a great choice, and they can actually improve your health since some of the iron makes its way into the food. They are inexpensive, and with proper care, they can be passed down for generations. You can put cast-iron pans into the oven, too, so they're versatile. You can also use stainless-steel cookware, which heats evenly and lasts a long time. It's what pro cooks use.

But how will you keep the food from sticking? The same way people have done for centuries: by using a little oil or water. If something sticks while cooking, you can unstick it by adding water and stirring the food to loosen the sticky parts. It takes but a few moments of time. In any case, you'll figure it out.

If you must keep using pans with nonstick surfaces:

+ Make sure they were manufactured after 2015, when PFAOs were forbidden.
+ Make sure they were made in the United States, since some foreign countries still allow PFAOs to be used.
+ Wash cookware gently with soap and water, and don't use metal utensils when cooking. If a pan gets chipped or scratched, toss it.
+ Don't heat a dry pan to the point where it begins to smoke, because the fumes it emits are a health hazard. In fact, here's what the official Teflon website has to say: "Avoid preheating nonstick pans on high heat without food in them—always start at a lower temperature using a fat like oil or butter or with the food already included. Empty pots and pans reach high temperatures very quickly, and when heated accidentally over 348 °C (660 °F) the coating can begin to deteriorate. . . . Do not use nonstick cookware and bakeware in ovens hotter than 260 °C (500 °F)."

Wow, even nonstick cookware needs to be greased with oil or fat. So what's the point of using it?

One final piece of advice: Replace nonstick cookware every few years. Or just skip using it altogether.

FATAL CONVENIENCES: AIR FRESHENERS

In the previous chapters, I talked a lot about the power of fragrance— how our brains are hard-wired to be disgusted by bad odors and mesmerized by good ones. For just about every species, the sense of smell is essential to survival. No wonder we can't help ourselves. Given that, are you surprised to learn that we in the United States spend somewhere in the neighborhood of $2 billion a year on products intended to make the air we inhale smell sweeter?

Are you shocked to find out that many of these products are harmful to our health? (Probably not at this point.) It makes sense that if we add a long list of toxic man-made chemicals to air that travels through our noses and into our lungs, we're asking for trouble. Yet that's exactly what we're doing when we spray air freshener into a room.

There's an amazing (or, depending on your point of view, crazy) array of products we use to perfume the air—sprays, gels, oils, liquids, solids, plug-ins, hanging disks, beads, potpourri, wick diffusers, scented candles; in active or passive forms; and with instant, intermittent, or continuous release. You can also go crazy and connect a fragrance diffuser to your home heating, ventilation, or air-conditioning system.

Air fresheners work in several ways. One is to capture the stinky molecules using something like cyclodextrin, a ring of starch derived from corn and potatoes that traps odors and locks them away, making them undetectable. These have lots of industrial uses as well. Odors can also be neutralized with citric acid, which regulates a smelly substance's pH.

In 1952, a passive air freshener was created when a dairy truck driver in upstate New York complained to the inventor Julius Sämann about the smell of spilled milk. To address the issue, Julius added pleasing fragrances to blotter material, inventing the first car air freshener. In honor of his years extracting aromatic oils in Canada's pine forests, he gave it the shape of an evergreen tree.

But when we think of air fresheners, we usually mean the big brands that simply mask strong scents by covering them up with even stronger scents. We all want our homes to smell like a pine forest, a grove of citrus trees, or freshly mown grass. Of course, it's too costly to make products using natural ingredients, so the smells are manufactured in industrial labs using synthesized chemicals. That's the convenience.

Naturally, there's a price to pay. Those sweet-smelling chemicals are now floating in a cloud all around you: on your skin, in your eyes, and, as I've already mentioned, infiltrating your respiratory system. Exposure to synthetic air fresheners, even at low levels, has been associated with a range of adverse health effects, including migraine headaches, asthma attacks, breathing difficulties, dermatitis, infant diarrhea and earaches, neurological problems, and ventricular fibrillation.

In 2007, the Natural Resources Defense Council (NRDC) published a paper showing that many air fresheners contain the hazardous chemicals phthalates, known to cause hormonal abnormalities, birth defects, and reproductive problems. Since then, some companies—but not all—have stopped using phthalates.

Researchers at the University of California, Berkeley, performed a study on air fresheners and household cleaners and discovered ethylene-based glycol ethers, classified by the EPA as hazardous pollutants. It also found the presence of terpenes, chemicals often derived from citrus oils that are not inherently dangerous except that they react with ozone in the air to form formaldehyde, which *is* toxic.

In fairness, the study reported that health issues apply mostly to professional cleaners who are exposed to high levels of these products. But as always, we have no idea how these chemicals react with all the other junk we inhale in the course of a normal day. So why subject ourselves to any more pollutants than we already do?

A chemical called 1,4-dichlorobenzene, which even moths are smart enough to avoid—it's present in mothballs—can also be found in some air fresheners. The EPA's air quality guide lists it as toxic since its vapors can affect respiratory function. The National Institute of Health Sciences has also reported that the chemicals in air fresheners can reduce lung capacity and may hasten respiratory diseases.

A University of Washington study found that eight unnamed, widely used air fresheners manufactured in the United States released an average of eighteen chemicals into the air. On average, one in five of the chemicals was a hazardous substance highlighted in federal and some state pollution standards. Half of the air fresheners tested released acetaldehyde, a likely human carcinogen according to the EPA.

Another University of Washington study of chemical hypersensitivity reported that around a third of participants who had asthma said that air fresheners aggravate their condition, and 40 percent reacted negatively to scented products in general.

Finally, as part of a 2009 study of cleaning supplies used in California schools, a total of eighty-nine airborne contaminants were detected, including acetaldehyde.

Included among the individual toxic chemicals in some of the most popular big-brand air fresheners are: cyclodextrin (can damage vision); dialkyl sulfosuccinates (can have reproductive system effects and cause skin allergies); sodium polyacrylate (is toxic to aquatic life, can cause respiratory damage); sodium sorbate (may reduce fertility); sodium borate (ditto); plus propane, isobutane, and the list goes on.

If you knew you were inhaling all those scary substances into your lungs, would you have been so hell-bent on perfuming the air you breathe? Do you believe that those chemical cocktails actually make your air *fresh*?

How About the Environment?

Just consider all the plastic spray bottles and cans being wasted on fairly useless products intended only to perfume (and pollute) the air we breathe. It's much wiser to eliminate the sources of bad smells than to poison ourselves trying to mask them.

Okay, So What Should We Do?

There are literally dozens of healthy, inexpensive do-it-yourself ways to rid your home of unpleasant smells and filling it with beautiful ones. They are listed in chapter 10, but here are a few good ideas.

Open some windows and turn on a fan or two. Or run the air conditioner. Maybe all you need to do is let some of the outdoors indoors and vice versa.

Fill a few containers with baking soda, which absorbs odors safely, and place them around your home.

Decorate with flowers, which can perfume any space. Plants are nice, too, but even though they recycle the air, you'd need a whole lot of them to make a difference in smells.

Fill a spray bottle with witch hazel, distilled water, and the essential oil of your choice and use it as an all-natural air freshener.

Buy or make a reed diffuser, fill it with a natural oil or other nontoxic fragrance.

Carbon and zeolite (a mineral) are used separately or together in filters for water, like in aquariums, but also to absorb bad air. Zeolite is especially effective against ammonia smells (think of your cat's litter box). Both of these are easily available online.

If you're really serious about smells, get an air purifier with a HEPA filter, which will remove allergens along with odors.

If you must use a commercial air freshener, buy one that discloses every ingredient, including whatever it uses for fragrance. And of course, make sure it does *not* contain any of the toxic chemicals we've just finished discussing.

On its website, the Environmental Working Group gives air fresheners letter grades from A to F that make it easy to find one that will do the job without making you and your family sick.

FATAL CONVENIENCES: PLASTIC FOOD STORAGE CONTAINERS

In theory, using food storage containers is a great idea. It probably means that you've cooked rather than ordered in, which is automatically an improvement in your nutritional health. If you're storing leftovers, it means that you're not wasting food, which is an enormous problem today. So far, so good. But what kind of containers are you using? If they're plastic, that's not so good.

I probably don't need to tell you what a chemist named Earl Tupper invented and began selling back in 1942. He used polyethylene slag, a smelly black waste product of oil refining, and turned it into plastic containers that he called "Welcome Ware." Later in the decade he added lids with a patented seal that closed with a "burp" to create a vacuum. With that innovation, Tupperware was born. It came along just as American homes began to have refrigerators large enough to store lots of food, making it possible for busy families to visit grocers weekly instead of daily.

Even before then, the first man-made plasticlike material was unveiled at the Second International Industrial Exhibition in London in 1862. It was derived from cellulose and was therefore plant based and biodegradable. It could be molded when heated and retained its shape when cooled. Too bad it didn't catch on.

The main health hazard of plastic food containers comes from what happens when they're heated. That's because heat releases the dangerous components of a toxic, hazardous, possibly hormone-disrupting chemical called bisphenol A, or BPA.

BPA is found in hardened plastic, meaning in water bottles, toys, and every kind of container, including the kind we use to store food and beverages. It's even in thermal paper receipts. Its molecules are held together by what's known to scientists as an ester bond, which is extremely sensitive to heat. When its temperature rises, the bonds break and the chemicals are unleashed. A survey by the CDC of 2,517 people estimated that more than 90 percent of Americans have detectable levels of BPA in their urine.

In 2018, the American Academy of Pediatrics expressed concern about scientific evidence showing that when bisphenols contaminate our food, they may interfere with hormones in ways that can affect children's long-term growth and development. BPA actually mimics estrogen and has been linked to reduced fertility in men and women, delayed puberty in girls, earlier puberty in boys, and behavioral problems in children.

In the same year, scientists at the University of California, San Francisco, found dozens of chemicals called environmental organic acids, or EOAs, in the blood of pregnant women. These chemicals, which include bisphenol A, have structures similar to that of hormones, meaning they may disrupt the endocrine system of a fetus and interfere with its development. Researchers involved in the study, which was published in the journal *Environmental Health Perspectives*, said that some of the chemicals had never before been documented in the blood of pregnant women, including two that are linked to genetic defects, fetal damage, and cancer. Among other chemicals detected was an estrogenic compound used in food-related plastic products, plastic pipes, and water bottles.

According to the Mayo Clinic, "Exposure to BPA is a concern because of the possible health effects on the brain and prostate gland of fetuses, infants and children. It can also affect children's behavior. Additional research suggests a possible link between BPA and increased blood pressure, type 2 diabetes and cardiovascular disease."

The evidence against BPA has been piling up over the past three decades. The EWG says that exposure to BPA may result in brain, behavioral, learning, and memory impairment, cardiovascular abnormalities, diabetes, obesity, breast and prostate cancer, thyroid and sex hormone disruption, early puberty, and changes to egg and sperm development and fertility. There's scary stuff in all that nice Tupperware, don't you think?

But even ridding products of BPA won't guarantee their safety. Research suggests that bisphenol S (BPS) and bisphenol F (BPF), the most common replacements, might have similar effects on the body. They are associated with obesity, particularly in children. According to a *Scientific American* article from 2014, "Nearly 81 percent of Americans have detectable levels of BPS in their urine. And once it enters the body it can affect cells in ways that parallel BPA." A 2013 study by researchers at the University of Texas found that even concentrations of less than one part per trillion of BPS can disrupt cells' normal functioning.

How About the Environment?

Look at it this way—single-use plastic, such as packaging and water bottles, is the scourge of our planet. Therefore, plastic that we reuse over and over has to be an improvement. And it is, except for the fact that at some point it will wear out and we'll toss it into the recycling bin, when it will join all the rest of the plastic junking up the world. In the end there's no kind of plastic that doesn't do long-term harm, these containers included. It's all toxic junk.

Okay, So What Should We Do?

You should use storage containers made of silicon rubber, stainless steel, glass, wood, ceramic, porcelain, or pretty much anything other than plastic. These are also safe if you reheat food in a microwave oven (except for metal containers, obviously), though you might want to reconsider that habit, too. Cutting as much plastic as possible from our lives is the safest way to go. Barring that:

Never heat anything in plastic.

Don't put plastic containers in your dishwasher, due to the high heat of the water in there.

Make sure food is cool before you store it in plastic.

Some families store pumped breast milk and baby formula in plastic containers—definitely a very bad idea!

Don't keep anything in plastic longer than necessary. The more time your food spends in contact with it, the greater the risk of contamination.

The smaller the container, the more of your food will be touching a plastic surface, so bigger is better.

Before you buy a plastic food storage container, check the bottom and avoid any with the recycling code 3, 6, or 7. They may contain phthalates, styrene, and bisphenols, unless they are labeled "biobased" or "greenware," indicating that they're made from corn and do not contain bisphenols.

FATAL CONVENIENCE: ALUMINUM FOIL, COOKWARE, AND CANS

Aluminum is the most abundant metal in the earth's crust, which explains the fact that it winds up in nearly all our food, water, soil, and air. Is it any surprise that your body contains some, too? The average American takes in around eight milligrams of aluminum every day, mostly through eating and drinking. How dangerous can it be? Give me a minute, and I'll get to that.

Going back to the Wright brothers, aluminum has been necessary to aviation; it's the only construction material sturdy enough but light enough to fly. Once somebody figured out how to roll the metal into thin sheets, it began to be used for wrapping fancy Swiss chocolates, chewing gum, mints, and other commercial products.

The first home use of aluminum foil began in the 1920s, but then, during World War II, people were encouraged to turn in their aluminum cookware and anything else made of aluminum, even foil from cigarette packs, to be recycled into war materials, as recycling the metal was cheaper than mining new supplies. Today, the global sales of aluminum foil total more than $24 billion—a lot of wrapping going on, mostly of edibles. It's really handy stuff, for both cooking as well as storing, and it looks pretty, too. That's where the nice part ends.

Since the 1960s, scientists have debated what they call "the aluminum hypothesis"—the possibility that aluminum found in the brain contributes to the development and progress of dementia. According to a 2011 paper published in the *International Journal of Alzheimer's Disease*, "it is widely accepted that Al [aluminum] is a recognized neurotoxin, and that it could cause cognitive deficiency and dementia when it enters the brain." So even though there's still no ironclad proof, there's definitely evidence of a link between metals and several brain diseases, such as amyotrophic lateral sclerosis (ALS, also known as Lou Gehrig's disease), dementia, and Parkinson's disease. As a neurotoxin, aluminum may slow the growth of brain cells—not a good thing. Those aren't the only potential hazards; it's also been linked to dialysis encephalopathy, bone disorders, and breast cancer.

Knowing all that, do you think that cutting back on your aluminum intake might be a good idea? Makes sense to me. Why take an unnecessary chance with the only brain you're ever going to get?

Our biggest exposure, beyond the environment, takes place in our kitchens. Research shows that food baked in aluminum foil contains more of the metal than when other kinds of cookware are used. If we're making foods high in acidity, such as tomato sauce, even more of it leaches into what we're about to eat. Salt also corrodes aluminum, meaning that there will be more metal in our meal. Still planning to barbecue using aluminum foil? *No bueno!*

How About the Environment?

Aluminum production is responsible for about 1.1 billion tons of CO_2 emissions per year, or roughly 2 percent of global emissions. But recycling cans and other objects uses only 5 percent as much energy. So recycling aluminum containers is better environmentally than owning any. But we're probably better off neither owning *nor* using new aluminum products.

Okay, What Should We Do?

It's impossible to avoid ingesting aluminum no matter what we try. But we can make a dent in the amount. Here are some tips for doing so.

Never cook, roast, bake, or steam anything in aluminum foil. I know, using foil makes cleanup easier, but this is a great example of a convenience that's not worth the cost. Lots of cooks wrap food in parchment paper before baking. Give that a try, but make sure you don't start an oven fire.

Don't use aluminum cookware if you can help it. If you must, make sure that the label says that it's either anodized or coated. Anodized means that it's been hardened through a process that renders the metal nonreactive. Coated means that it's been clad in stainless steel or ceramic, so the metal itself doesn't touch your food. If the pan is neither anodized nor coated, you and your family are having a side dish of aluminum along with whatever else you're eating.

Needless to say, drinking out of aluminum cans also seems like a bad idea, not to mention the fact that it's rare to find a healthy beverage that is sold in cans (even though beer *is* a plant-based product).

FATAL CONVENIENCES: BEDS AND BEDDING

We spend around a third of our lives lying in bed, totally out of it, completely vulnerable, believing that at least during those precious hours we're safe from harm. Sweet dreams.

Experts keep reminding us how important it is to our mental and physical health to get plenty of high-quality sleep. It regulates our blood sugar, reduces stress, enhances our immune system, and provides a long list of other benefits. The reality is that your face is buried in a pillow made of synthetic materials you probably haven't bothered to research, and the rest of you is nestled in sheets, blankets, and comforters containing man-made fibers and fabrics just as unknown to you—and I'm guessing not as safe as you might imagine.

Early beds, from the dawn of humankind until some point in the twentieth century, were made of natural materials, because that was all that existed: straw, wood, bamboo, reeds, wool, animal skins, feathers, cotton, linen. Whether they were organic or not wasn't a consideration because there was no widespread use of pesticides. Often, sheets were woven on looms at home.

Bedding today is a whole other thing. Your mattress contains lots of substances you're not aware of, including dust and the tiny bugs— dust mites—that feed on it, plus your discarded dead skin and hair cells, plus various assorted fungi, and so on. That's slightly disgusting to think about, though not lethal.

But your bedding was probably manufactured and treated with a long list of industrial chemicals and nonnatural substances. A main reason is cost; synthetic fibers are cheaper to make than plant-based ones are to grow, harvest, and process. Then there are the superpowers that I mentioned in the chapter on clothing: material that never wrinkles, never stains, never burns, and may even be able to resist bacteria.

As helpful as all those features sound, each brings negatives, which usually outweigh the positives. I've already talked about the flame-retardant scam in the entry on furniture, but to recap: these are dangerous chemicals that off-gas into our lungs and have been linked to everything from cancer and endocrine-system disruption to allergies. Plus, they're not really much good at fighting fires. Even with all that, for a while government agencies were forcing manufacturers of mattresses and furniture to treat their products with this junk. If you've ever bought a new mattress and noticed that odd, unnatural "new bed" smell, you were inhaling flame-retardant gas.

Your pillows are probably not any safer. Most nowadays are made with synthetic materials, small plastic beads or polyester, including a chemical called ethylene glycol. It can cause allergic reactions, skin irritation, nausea, and respiratory depression. Memory foam pillows are made from polyurethane, which shows up in most furniture, too. It off-gasses volatile organic compounds (VOCs) that we breathe into our noses and lungs. Our kids and pets inhale them, too.

Formaldehyde, benzidine, parathion, and mercury are all part of the manufacturing process of the cotton used in sheets and bedding and can potentially remain part of the fabric.

Blended-fabric sheets and other bedding—meaning cotton-polyester mixtures—are still partly petroleum based, with all the toxicity that comes with that. And the cotton for standard-issue sheets was grown using pesticides, meaning that they're harmful to the environment and not so great for you, either.

Wrinkle-free sheets have the same dangers as no-iron clothing does. The resins used in their manufacture contain formaldehyde, which can cause dermatitis, throat irritation, and nausea. But that's not all; in 1987, the EPA classified formaldehyde as a probable human carcinogen. Then, in 2011, the National Toxicology Program stepped that up, calling it a known human carcinogen. It's better to live with wrinkled sheets (or learn to iron).

How About the Environment?

Bedding fabrics create the same problems as do all the fabrics I've discussed in this book. Nonorganic cotton comes with a huge environmental cost, from the water needed to grow and process it to pesticides and GMOs to chemical treatments to the nonbiodegradable polyester content. Discarded mattresses, blankets, pillows, and sheets pile up in landfills somewhere, poisoning the earth, which in turn contaminates the water below.

Okay, So What Should We Do?

Choose sheets, blankets, comforters, and pillows made using natural fibers only, meaning organic cotton, linen, silk, and wool. Even some offbeat materials such as kapok, buckwheat, millet, and other plant-based fibers are now being used. Not only are these safer to have against your face and body, but they breathe, so your skin can, too. And they'll wick away moisture better than synthetic fibers do. The downside is that they're more expensive than the other kinds. Organic cotton sheets can cost double or even triple the conventional ones. But what you spend today will benefit your health for years to come. Avoid blended materials such as cotton or silk mixed with polyester and other synthetics—even satin sheets, sorry to tell you adventurous sleepers. As with clothing, don't buy bedding with wrinkle-free, antistatic, or any other superpowers.

Today, shopping for mattresses is more complicated than ever due to all the choices and the confusing terminology. Our best bet, as always, is to stick with natural materials, such as organic cotton and organic wool. If you're really worried about your bed going up in flames, either stop smoking there or invest in a mattress made of wool, which is naturally fire resistant. Be wary of something called a fire sock, which is a flame-resistant covering made of fiberglass or other synthetic materials.

Look for bedding with a Global Organic Textile Standard (GOTS) label. This certification means that at least 70 percent of the fibers are organic and that ethical treatment of workers and environmentally friendly manufacturing standards are in place.

9

SOME FINAL THOUGHTS

I'VE THROWN A LOT OF INFORMATION at you in these pages, but I've only scratched the surface. When you consider the sheer number of toxic substances out there, you realize how impossible it would be for anyone to keep track of them all. Every day, new studies come out detailing just how hazardous modern life has become.

Aside from all the particulars of the Fatal Conveniences, one message I've tried to get across is this: We all need to be extremely careful about everything we buy and use and consume. As I said back at the beginning, we need to interrogate each product in our lives. We need to ask: What exactly *are* you? What do you contain? What do you do to make my life better? Do I really need you at all? And what *aren't* you telling me on the front package label that you divulge only on the back in print so tiny it's illegible, in words that are meaningless to anyone but a scientist? We need to get straight answers to those questions.

We go through life assuming that if something can legally be sold, it must be harmless. If it's in a drugstore, it must be healthy. If it's in a grocery store, it must be safe to eat. If it comes out of the kitchen tap, it must be okay to drink. We are woefully wrong in those assumptions. In fact, that halo of wholesomeness is what deceives us into dropping our guard and consuming things that do us harm.

But hang on a second—can't we rely on government agencies at the federal, state, county, and local levels to protect us from things that will make us sick and shorten our lives? They wouldn't allow toxic substances to be sold, would they?

They would.

Not because those bureaucracies, administrations, and boards wish us ill, but because there's no way they can keep up with all the hazards in the world today. And also because when government comes up against big business, you can guess who usually wins. Sad to say, it's in the corporate world's best interests to keep pumping out products that are bad for our health and to keep pouring pollutants into our environment. It's the capitalist way. We have put the god of profit ahead of our health.

But there are countermeasures that can be taken, and lucrative ones at that. We can help by consuming in our best (health) interests.

We live in fear of getting cancer and wonder why no cure has been discovered despite the fortune we spend on research. But then we use consumer products containing chemicals that are proven carcinogens, relying on government agencies' assurances that their levels are too low to harm us and forgetting how many times in the past such assurances have been proven false.

Or we go around saying "Men are producing dramatically less sperm than they once did, and birthrates are falling, oh, what could be behind this scary situation?" Meanwhile, fetuses are absorbing one proven endocrine-system disruptor after another, chemicals that we *know* have a damaging effect on our ability to reproduce.

Hello? Are we suicidal? Do we really not understand that those chemicals might be to blame and maybe we ought to quit using them? Or is it just that we'd rather keep putting toxic substances into our bodies even if it means we'll never have grandchildren?

A lot of my thinking about Fatal Conveniences can be explained by a concept known as *allostatic load*, a scientific term for a fairly simple idea: that all the chemicals and other substances we're exposed to on a daily basis have a cumulative effect on our health that's impossible to measure. There are just too many things going on on too many different levels for scientists to determine the total impact on our bodies.

There's a related term: *allostatic overload*. You can probably guess what that one means, but I'll quote the abstract of a survey that examined the results of 267 original studies: "Allostatic load refers to the cumulative burden of chronic stress and life events. It involves the interaction of different physiological systems at varying degrees of activity. When environmental challenges exceed the individual ability to cope, then allostatic overload ensues."

One sentence there needs to be repeated: "When environmental challenges exceed the individual ability to cope, then allostatic overload ensues." That's where we are today: in overload. This is why all the assurances that chemicals are harmless in the amounts we ingest are worthless. This is the reason all the promises that the radiation from our digital devices won't damage our DNA are deceptive. Because we're not getting just a few chemicals, we're getting thousands. We're not absorbing just a small amount of radiation, we're bathed in it twenty-four hours a day.

No scientist, no researcher has ever figured out how to measure the effects of all that on every human body. Even the combined powers of the FDA, the EPA, the CDC, Procter & Gamble, Maybelline, General Foods, and Apple can't tell you how the total onslaught of supposedly "safe" chemicals and radiation will affect your health.

AS I'VE BEEN WORKING ON this book, I've also been shooting a series for Netflix called *Down to Earth*. While doing that, I've been immersed in solutions big and small to our planet's problems. I've been introduced to companies such as Footprint (footprintus.com), a B-to-B outfit creating alternatives to single-use plastic. It's now working with nine of the top ten consumer goods corporations in the world, including Walmart, McDonald's, and Conagra Brands. Maybe someday the tidal wave of plastic that has engulfed us will no longer exist.

By now we've all heard and read the words *climate crisis* a million times. Experts, politicians, government officials, and activists tell us to do this or stop doing that "because of climate change." We get a nonstop stream of lectures about how our habits and consumer choices are damaging something called "the environment."

I get it. I totally do. But I had a sudden realization, like a bolt of lightning: the way we think about this subject is a big part of the problem. We've been taught to think of "the environment" as something separate from ourselves. As though the environment is out there, in terrible danger, but we're in here, safe and sound. To some people, that may be a comforting thought. But it's not true. We're all part of the environment, the same as every tree, lake, fish, and flower. We're just one more living thing, with the same basic needs as every other creature. If something damages the planet, it damages each of us as an individual. If I drink a plastic bottle of water, I'm being poisoned by all the chemicals, phthalates, petrochemicals, endocrine disruptors, and other garbage in it. Once I finish the water and throw the bottle away, the bottle poisons the world outside my body. Then that pollution comes back and poisons me again. This is the cycle we've created. As long as I can think of the environment as something separate from my own body, I can kid myself into thinking that I'm safe. Except I'm not. If it hurts me, it hurts the environment. If it hurts the environment, it hurts me. We're one and the same.

The "crisis" isn't just about the climate up in the atmosphere. It's right here in the choices we make and the way we live. Every convenience we purchase either harms us or helps us. If we choose healthy products, we and our planet will both benefit. Keep that in mind next time you shop for food, toothpaste, a mattress, a T-shirt, or anything else. Wake up, take action, enjoy every nonfatal convenience, and live your best life ever— your superlife!

10

OKAY, SO *NOW* WHAT SHOULD WE DO?

WE'D ALL LOVE EVERYTHING WE BUY and use to be natural, healthy, and green. But when those buzzwords become trendy, it's a mixed blessing. On the one hand, it means we have more options and can find safe products even at little local shops and big chain stores. But it also creates the deceptive marketing practice known as "greenwashing," coined by the environmentalist Jay Westerveld in 1986.

He chided hotels for touting how environmentally sensitive they were for reusing towels, while simultaneously engaging in other practices that were far worse. Since then, the term has been widely used to expose brands that spend lots of effort on advertising and packaging their products as clean and natural—without investing in practices that make their merchandise less harmful to you and me.

So as you go through life trying to find products that won't make you sick and kill you, don't get sucked in by the sales pitch. Here are some good brands you can try and reliable sources of useful information, along with the ultimate in Safe Conveniences: products you can make yourself.

PERSONAL CARE PRODUCTS

Deodorant

DIY Deodorant No. 1

2½ tablespoons unrefined coconut oil (suggested: Carrington Farms Organic Coconut Oil)

2½ tablespoons unrefined shea butter (suggested: Taha Natural Shea Butter)

¼ cup arrowroot starch or flour (suggested: Bob's Red Mill Arrowroot Starch)

1½ tablespoons baking soda

6 drops lavender essential oil (suggested: Aura Cacia 100% Pure Lavender Essential Oil)

6 drops grapefruit essential oil

1 drop tea tree essential oil

Place the coconut oil and shea butter in a glass bowl or jar and place the bowl or jar inside a medium saucepan. Add enough water to the saucepan to surround the bowl or jar without overflowing into it and bring it to a boil.

Stir the coconut oil and shea butter continuously until they melt.

Once they are melted, remove pan from the heat and add the arrowroot starch, baking soda, and essential oils.

Pour into a 3-ounce glass jar, cover, and cool at room temperature or in the fridge until it reaches a solid state.

Source: *Healthy Maven (thehealthymaven.com)*

DIY Deodorant No. 2

¼ teaspoon Himalayan salt or sea salt

6 drops lemon essential oil (suggested: Aura Cacia Lemon Essential Oil)

1 drop geranium essential oil (suggested: Aura Cacia Geranium
   Essential Oil)
2 tablespoons rosewater
2 tablespoons grain alcohol, Everclear, or high-proof vodka
   (don't use rubbing alcohol because you can become sensi-
   tized to it with regular use)
4 tablespoons pure witch hazel (suggested: WH Witch Hazel,
   100% Natural Astringent)

Combine the salt and essential oils in a small spray bottle and gently shake to combine.

Using a funnel, add the rosewater, alcohol, and witch hazel. Tighten
the cap and shake.

Spray onto clean armpits and allow to dry briefly before dressing.

Source: *Kitchn (thekitchn.com)*

Sources of Vegan/Nontoxic Deodorants

+ **Native:** Durable protection, clean, and free of the nasties
  (nativecos.com)
+ **Tom's of Maine:** Twenty-four-hour wetness and odor protection
  made entirely of ingredients derived from plants and minerals
  (tomsofmaine.com)
+ **Aubrey Organics:** Natural herbal extracts without harsh ingredients or preservatives (available at pureformulas.com)
+ **Desert Essence:** Made with antibacterial botanical extracts and essential oils; aluminum free (desertessence.com)
+ **Dr. Hauschka:** A roll-on with no aluminum salts (drhauschka.com)
+ **EcoRoots:** Clean, nontoxic, natural deodorant; aluminum free,
  paraben free, cruelty free, baking soda free, and vegan (www
  .ecoroots.us)
+ **Ethique bars:** Vegan, palm oil free, cruelty free, aluminum free, and
  nontoxic (available at amazon.com)

+ **NaturisticBath:** Vegan and formulated without artificial or synthetic ingredients, aluminum, and baking soda (NaturisticBath at etsy.com)
+ **Meow Meow Tweet:** A US-made zero-waste deodorant brand that is vegan and palm oil free (meowmeowtweet.com)
+ **Hammond Herbs:** Free from aluminum, parabens, synthetic preservatives, synthetic fragrances, and animal testing (hammond herbs.com)

Sources of Refillable Deodorants

+ **Nuud:** Free from aluminum, artificial fragrances, and alcohol (nuudcare.com)
+ **By Humankind:** All initial purchases of deodorant and mouthwash come in refillable, recyclable containers with a lifetime guarantee. (byhumankind.com)
+ **Lush:** Packaging-free options (www.lushusa.com)
+ **Wild:** Product cases are customizable and made with anodized aluminum and recycled plastic. All refills are 100 percent plastic free. No parabens, artificial fragrances, or aluminum. The company also contributes a percentage of its sales to the reforestation charity On a Mission. (wearewild.com)

For more information on cruelty-free deodorant, check out the PETA Certified List (crueltyfree.peta.org/product-type/?product=deodorant).

Toothpaste

DIY Toothpaste No. 1

8 tablespoons sodium bicarbonate (cleans with its abrasive
  properties and neutralizes stains and odors)
6 tablespoons glycerin (is both a lubricant and a binder)

10–15 drops peppermint oil (adds the taste we all associate with a fresh mouth)

1 drop clove oil (is antimicrobial, antiviral, and antifungal)

Mix all ingredients in a glass jar with a lid and use within two months.

Source: *Lindsay Miles (treadingmyownpath.com)*

DIY Toothpaste No. 2

2 tablespoons baking soda

2 tablespoons coconut oil

10 drops essential oil (use your favorite)

Mix all ingredients in a glass jar with a lid and use within two months.

Natural and Organic Toothpastes

+ **Lebon Organic Toothpaste:** Contains organic aloe vera and green tea to help prevent gum disease and tooth decay. With natural flavors such as pineapple, rooibos, mint, rose, and orange blossom. (lebonandlebon.com)
+ **Bite Toothpaste Bits:** Clean, safe product in sustainable packaging (bitetoothpastebits.com; use discount code DARIN20)
+ **Dr. Bronner's All-One Toothpaste:** Vegan and mint flavored (drbronner.com)
+ **Tom's of Maine Cavity Protection Natural Toothpaste:** Not tested on animals and has no artificial flavors, colors, or preservatives (tomsofmaine.com)
+ **Himalaya Neem and Pomegranate Toothpaste:** Cruelty free (himalayausa.com)
+ **ETEE Chewpaste:** Formulated with Canadian glacial clay, kaolin clay, and sodium laurel sulfoacetate, it contains no sulfates and is vegan and cruelty free. The product comes in a glass jar with a steel

lid. When empty, you can purchase more of the refillable toothpaste in compostable pouches. (shopetee.com)

+ **Georganics Natural Mineral-Rich Toothpaste:** Eco friendly with no fluoride, SLS, palm oil, or glycerin. Contains calcium carbonate and sodium bicarbonate, which reduce tooth sensitivity. (georganics.com)

+ **The Dirt Trace Mineral Tooth Brushing Powder:** Vegan, paleo, and free from fluoride, glycerin, and GMO-derived xylitol (givemethedirt.com)

+ **Scentcerae Tooth Nibs:** Little nuggets that you place inside your mouth, chew, and then brush normally. Contain bentonite clay, white kaolin clay, illite sea clay, sodium bicarbonate, natural soap nuts, and organic xylitol. (scentcerae.com)

An Alternative to Traditional Oral Care

+ **Oil pulling:** This technique has been used for centuries. You just take a tablespoon or so of oil into your mouth—you can use olive oil, but I prefer coconut—and swish it around like mouthwash for 10 to 20 minutes before spitting it out. The oil picks up the bacteria, viruses, and other junk from your teeth, tongue, and gums, leaving your mouth clean and bad microbe free. Your dentist might never have heard of this, but there are plenty of scientific studies proving that it works.

Foods That Help Keep Teeth Healthy

+ **Celery, carrots, and other crunchy veggies:** These foods, which contain lots of fiber, are natural cleaners because they stimulate saliva flow, which scrubs away food particles and bacteria while neutralizing citric and malic acids.

+ **Leafy greens (spinach, kale, lettuce, and others):** These are rich in calcium, folic acids, minerals, and vitamins that are beneficial for teeth.

+ **Apples and pears:** The fiber in these fruits increases saliva flow.
+ **Nuts:** These are packed with calcium and phosphorus, which help fight decay.

Source: *University of Illinois Chicago College of Dentistry (dentistry.uic.edu)*

Sunscreen

DIY Sunscreen

¼ cup coconut oil (has a natural SPF of 7)
25 drops walnut extract oil for scent and an added SPF boost
1 cup shea butter for consistency
¼ cup pure aloe vera gel (recommended: Bioactif Pure Aloe Vera Gel)
2 tablespoons powdered zinc oxide (or more if you like)

In a medium saucepan over medium heat, combine all ingredients except the aloe vera gel and the zinc oxide. Stir and let everything melt together.

Let cool for several minutes before stirring in the aloe vera gel.

Cool completely before adding the zinc oxide. Mix well to make sure the zinc oxide is distributed throughout.

Store in a glass jar, and keep in a cool, dry place until ready to use.

Two caveats:

- This solution is not waterproof, so it must be reapplied frequently if used in a pool or at the beach.
- For oily skin, swap jojoba or sweet almond oil for the coconut oil.

Source: *Kathryn Watson (healthline.com)*

Safe Sunscreens

- **Banana Boat Sport Mineral Lotion SPF 50+:** This sunscreen provides a high endurance-versus-sweat ratio and 100 percent mineral composition. It's great for sensitive skin and free from potentially harmful chemicals such as oxybenzone, parabens, and phthalates. It has the National Eczema Association seal of acceptance. (bananaboat.com)

- **Banana Boat Sensitive 100% Mineral Lotion SPF 50+:** Formulated with naturally sourced zinc, it's hypoallergenic and has a National Eczema Association seal of acceptance. Zinc oxide and titanium dioxide are the only active ingredients, with no added oils or fragrances. Also recommended by the Skin Cancer Foundation. (bananaboat.com)

- **Babo Botanicals Baby Skin Mineral Sunscreen:** This might be more expensive than the other options mentioned, but its formula is hypoallergenic and rated number one in safety by the Environment Working Group (EWG). Made from 100 percent mineral zinc for broad spectrum UVA and UVB protection. (babobotanicals.com)

- **Sun Bum Moisturizing Sunscreen Lotion:** Protects against UVA and UVB rays and is water resistant for up to eighty minutes. Tested and approved by the Skin Cancer Foundation; suitable for all skin types; paraben free, oil free, hypoallergenic, gluten free, noncomedogenic, reef friendly, dermatologist approved, octinoxate free, and oxybenzone free. (sunbum.com)

- **Suntegrity Sunscreen:** Non−nano zinc oxide and titanium dioxide. Other ingredients include grapeseed oil, karanja oil, squalane, argan oil, olive oil, papaya and mango fruit extracts, and rice bran extract. Nonaerosol and TSA-friendly size. (suntegrityskincare.com)

- **Babo Botanicals Daily Sheer Fluid SPF 50 Tinted Sunscreen:** Non−nano zinc oxide mineral sunscreen combined with sweet white lupine for broad-spectrum SPF 50 protection against UVA, UVB, and blue light. Fragrance free and suitable for all skin types, although it is especially good for sensitive skin. Rich in vitamins and antioxidants. (babobotanicals.com)

+ **Babo Botanicals Sheer Mineral Sunscreen SPF 50:** Formulated for all sensitive skin types; provides eighty minutes of water and sweat resistance (babobotanicals.com)

+ **Lumiton:** A clothing brand whose garments convert harmful UV rays into red and near-infrared light, bathing you in healthy frequencies (lumiton.com)

Tips from the Skin Cancer Foundation

+ Limit your sun exposure between 10:00 a.m. and 4:00 p.m., even in winter.

+ Remember that trees, umbrellas, and hats provide imperfect protection.

+ Snow, water, and sand are powerful reflectors of the sun's rays, so be extra careful in their presence.

+ Clothing provides some protection depending on a number of factors. Intense colors absorb UV rays better than light-colored garments do. If you can see light through the fabric, it won't be much protection from the sun. Keep the following factors in mind when shopping.

  ~ **Color:** Dark or bright colors keep UV rays from reaching your skin by absorbing them.

  ~ **Construction:** Densely woven cloth, such as denim, canvas, wool, or synthetic fiber, is more protective than sheer, thin, or loosely woven cloth.

  ~ **Tip:** Check a fabric's sun safety by holding it up to the light. If you can see through it, UV radiation can easily penetrate the fabric and reach your skin.

  ~ **Content:** Unbleached cotton contains natural lignans that act as UV absorbers. Shiny polyesters and even lightweight satiny silks can be highly protective because they reflect radiation. High-tech fabrics treated with chemical UV absorbers.

~ **Fit:** Loose-fitting apparel is preferable. Tight clothing can stretch and reduce the level of protection offered.

~ **UPF:** Some clothing makers provide ultraviolet protection factor (UPF) labels that indicate exactly how much of the sun's rays the garment can shield.

~ **Coverage:** The more skin your outfit covers, the better. Whenever possible, wear long-sleeved shirts and long pants or skirts.

Source: *The Skin Cancer Foundation (skincancer.org)*

Moisturizer

DIY Moisturizer No. 1

2 1/2 ounces avocado, apricot, jojoba, almond, or other oil
2 1/2 ounces shea, coconut, mango, or cocoa butter
1/2 ounce beeswax (hard shavings are best)
3 1/2 ounces distilled water
25 drops grapefruit seed extract
20 drops essential oil of your choice

Mix all ingredients in a glass jar with a lid.

Source: *Bellatory (bellatory.com)*

DIY Moisturizer No. 2

3/4 cup aloe vera gel
1/4 cup distilled or purified water
1/2 cup beeswax, grated or pellets
1/2 cup jojoba or sweet almond oil
1 teaspoon vitamin E oil
15 drops lavender essential oil (optional)

Mix all ingredients in a glass jar with a lid.

Source: *Treehugger (treehugger.com)*

Sources of Nontoxic Moisturizers

+ **Caldera + Lab** (calderalab.com)
+ **Kora Organics** (us.koraorganics.com)
+ **Mad Hippie** (madhippie.com)
+ **Amazon Aware** (amazon.com)
+ **Avalon Organics** (avalonorganics.com)
+ **True Botanicals** (truebotanicals.com)
+ **Inna Organic** (innaorganic.co)
+ **Mineral Fusion** (mineralfusion.com)
+ **The Earthling Co.** (theearthlingco.com)
+ **Cocokind** (cocokind.com)
+ **Primally Pure** (primallypure.com)
+ **100% Pure** (100percentpure.com)
+ **Dr. Bronner's** (drbronner.com)
+ **Biossance** (biossance.com)
+ **OSEA** (oseamalibu.com)
+ **Prima** (prima.co)
+ **The Honest Company** (honest.com)

Additional Resources

+ **EWG's Skin Deep:** Has excellent information to help you choose safe and green products (ewg.org/skindeep/)
+ **Think Dirty:** Another good source of information (thinkdirty app.com)
+ **Yuka:** Yet another good source of information (yuka.io)

Soap and Bodywash

DIY Bodywash No. 1

2/3 cup liquid Castile soap

1/4 cup raw honey

2 teaspoons jojoba oil (you can also use sweet almond, grape-
    seed, sesame, or olive oil)
1 teaspoon vitamin E oil
50–60 drops essential oil of your choice

Mix all ingredients in a glass bottle.

Source: *DIY Natural (diynatural.com)*

DIY Bodywash No. 2

½ cup shea butter
1 tablespoon apricot oil
1 tablespoon aloe vera gel
2 tablespoons vegetable glycerin
3 drops spearmint essential oil
6 drops bergamot essential oil
3 drops vetiver essential oil
1 cup liquid Castile soap

Mix all ingredients in a 16-ounce pump dispenser bottle.

Source: *DIY Natural (diynatural.com)*

Sources of Safe Soap and Bodywash

- **Caldera + Lab** (calderalab.com)
- **Kora Organics** (us.koraorganics.com)
- **Mad Hippie** (madhippie.com)
- **Amazon Aware** (amazon.com)
- **Avalon Organics** (avalonorganics.com)
- **True Botanicals** (truebotanicals.com)
- **Inna Organic** (innaorganic.co)
- **Mineral Fusion** (mineralfusion.com)
- **The Earthling Co.** (theearthlingco.com)
- **Cocokind** (cocokind.com)

+ **Primally Pure** (primallypure.com)
+ **100% Pure** (100percentpure.com)
+ **Dr. Bronner's** (drbronner.com)
+ **Biossance** (biossance.com)
+ **OSEA** (oseamalibu.com)
+ **Prima** (prima.co)
+ **The Honest Company** (honest.com)

Fragrances

Each of these perfumes requires a glass roller, a carrier oil (such as jojoba, sweet almond, or grapeseed oil), and 100 percent essential oil for scent. All recipes are from Hello Glow (helloglow.co).

DIY Floral Perfume

1 ounce carrier oil
5 drops sweet orange essential oil
2 drops organic lime essential oil
2 drops jasmine absolute in jojoba oil
2 drops vanilla in jojoba oil

Mix all ingredients in a glass jar or bottle with a lid.

DIY Rose Perfume

1 ounce carrier oil
2 drops rose absolute essential oil
4 drops sandalwood in jojoba oil
5 drops bergamot essential oil

Mix all ingredients in a glass jar or bottle with a lid.

DIY Citrus Perfume

1 ounce carrier oil
2 drops lemon essential oil

3 drops lime essential oil
5 drops vanilla in jojoba oil

Mix all ingredients in a glass jar or bottle with a lid.

How to Choose an Essential Oil

+ **Woody scent:** Cedarwood, pine, or labdanum
+ **Musky scent:** Botanical musk or ambrette
+ **Citrus scent:** Bergamot, lemon, or grapefruit
+ **Herbal scent:** Lavender, chamomile, or rosemary
+ **Floral scent:** Rose, geranium, iris, jasmine, magnolia, peony, or ylang-ylang

Sources of Safe Fragrances

+ **Tsila Organics:** Perfume oils (tsilaorganics.com)
+ **Eden's Garden:** Essential oil perfumes (edensgarden.com)
+ **1912 Aromatherapy:** Aromatherapy products (1912aroma therapy.com)
+ **Doterra:** Essential oils (doterra.com)

Perfume oils are a good alternative to liquid and spray perfumes; they're often made of cleaner ingredients and also last longer.

Cosmetics

DIY Lipstick

1 teaspoon beeswax pellets
1 teaspoon shea, cocoa, or mango butter
1–2 teaspoons sweet almond or coconut oil
1/8 teaspoon beetroot powder

Place the beeswax, butter, and oil in the top of a double boiler, glass liquid measuring cup, or heatproof bowl. Put the bowl or measuring cup in a saucepan filled halfway with water. Bring the water to a simmer. Let it simmer until the mixture is melted.

Remove from heat and mix in any additional ingredients for color or scent.

Use a dropper to quickly transfer the liquid into a small jar. Allow a bit of room at the top since the mixture will expand slightly as it cools.

Cool for at least 30 minutes or until completely hardened before putting on the lid.

Store in a dry, cool place. Use within 6 months.

Source: *Healthline (healthline.com)*

Sources of Safe Cosmetics

+ **ZeroWasteStore:** Discloses all ingredients and offers refillable makeup products (zerowastestore.com)
+ **Neek Skin Organics:** A vegan, cruelty-free makeup brand that uses sustainable packaging and is free from synthetic dyes, parabens, phthalates, sulfates, mineral oil, palm oil, perfume, and lead (neekskinorganics.com)
+ **The Clean Beauty Box:** May be best known for its monthly prescription boxes, but to reduce waste, consider buying only its individual products (cleanbeautybox.com)
+ **RMS Beauty:** One of the oldest clean beauty brands (rms beauty.com)

Additional Resources

Good Face Project: Analyzes and rates cosmetic ingredients (thegood faceproject.com)

Shampoo and Conditioner

DIY Shampoo Bar

1 cup melt-and-pour Castile soap base
1 teaspoon olive oil
1/2 teaspoon castor oil
1/2 teaspoon black molasses
15 drops vanilla essential oil
15 drops patchouli essential oil
10 drops rosemary essential oil

Cut the melt-and-pour soap base into small cubes. Add to a double boiler or an aluminum bowl in a pan half filled with warm water over low to medium heat. The water should be simmering, not boiling. Stir continuously until the soap base is melted.

Add the olive oil, castor oil, and black molasses and mix well.

Take the bowl off the heat and wait a few minutes until slightly cooled.

Add the essential oils and mix well.

Pour into a soap mold and let harden for 24 hours. No need to store.

Source: *Healthline (healthline.com)*

Online Sources of Safe Shampoo and Conditioner

+ **Dr. Bronner's** (also available in stores) (drbronner.com)
+ **True Botanicals** (truebotanicals.com)
+ **Ceremonia** (ceremonia.com)
+ **100% Pure** (100percentpure.com)
+ **Ursa Major** (ursamajorvt.com)
+ **Zero Waste** (zerowastestore.com)
+ **Puracy** (puracy.com)

Safe Shampoo and Conditioner Brands Sold in Stores

+ Herbal Essences Bio:Renew Sulfate-Free Shampoo
+ Pipette Nourishing Shampoo

Additional Resources

As I said earlier, the entire personal care category is a minefield of hazardous products. Fortunately, the Environmental Working Group has a program to verify safe, environmentally sane products that meet its strict, scientific standards for transparency and health. That means that the products don't contain any ingredients causing health, ecotoxicity, or contamination concerns and the manufacturers are transparent about all the ingredients on their labels, including fragrance, and follow good manufacturing practices. The EWG has also created a database of personal care products on which you can check their ingredients against a list of regulatory databases and see whether their manufacturers test on animals. These evaluations can be found at ewg.org/skindeep. You can look for the EWG Verified label on products sold in stores, too.

The nonprofit Nontoxic Certified created the MADE SAFE seal to verify the personal care products that don't contain any of the 6,500 substances on its banned list. It also looks for products that will not harm our water, air, and soil. You can find info at madesafe.org or look for the MADE SAFE seal on product labels.

FOODS AND BEVERAGES

Fast Foods

Plant-Based/Organic "Fast-Food" (but Not the Evil Kind) Restaurant Chains

+ **Grabbagreen** (grabbagreen.com)
+ **Sweetgreen** (sweetgreen.com)
+ **Freshii** (freshii.com)
+ **Veggie Grill** (veggiegrill.com)

Dairy Products

When making DIY nut milk, a nut milk machine such as Nutr (thenutr .com) or Almond Cow (almondcow.co) simplifies the process.

DIY Pistachio Milk

1 cup dry pistachio nuts
4 cups filtered water

Soak the nuts for six hours or overnight. You can then peel them for a brighter green pistachio milk, but this isn't necessary.

Place the soaked nuts into a high-speed food processor or blender and blend on high. You want to break them down into small pieces without turning them into pistachio butter.

When the nuts are ready, add the water and blend again for about 1–2 minutes.

Pour into a large glass bottle (you can use a nut milk bag if you have one) and store in the fridge up to 3 to 5 days. Shake well before drinking.

Source: *Alpha Foodie (alphafoodie.com)*

DIY Oat Milk

1/2 cup whole rolled oats (organic)

3 cups water

2 teaspoons maple syrup (or stevia or monkfruit sweetener)

1/2 teaspoon vanilla extract

1/8 teaspoon sea salt

Combine the oats, water, maple syrup, vanilla, and salt in a blender and blend for 30 seconds.

Place a fine mesh strainer over a large bowl and strain the milk without pushing any excess pulp through the strainer. This will create a creamy texture that's not gritty or gummy.

Add more maple syrup to taste, if desired. Chill overnight. If you want to drink the oat milk right away, I recommend adding ice, as it tastes best when chilled.

Source: *Love and Lemons (loveandlemons.com)*

DIY Vegan Cheese Sauce

3/4 cup peeled and diced Yukon Gold potato

3/4 cup peeled and diced sweet potato

2 garlic cloves

1/4 cup raw cashews

1 tablespoon apple cider vinegar

2 tablespoons nutritional yeast

1/2 teaspoon onion powder

1/2 teaspoon sea salt

1/4 cup extra-virgin olive oil

1/4 cup water

To make the cheese spicy or smoky, add:

1/2–1 chipotle pepper from canned chipotles in adobo

1 tablespoon pickled jalapeños

1/4–1/2 teaspoon smoked paprika

Place the potatoes in a saucepan and cover with cold water by about 1 inch. Add a few pinches of salt. Bring to a boil, then reduce the heat and simmer, uncovered, until fork tender, 8 to 12 minutes.

Drain and transfer to a high-speed blender. Add the garlic, cashews, vinegar, nutritional yeast, onion powder, salt, olive oil, and ¼ cup water. Blend until smooth.

For spicy vegan cheese, add the chipotle pepper or pickled jalapeños. For a smoky flavor, add the smoked paprika.

Serve with tortilla chips for dipping or over pasta to make vegan mac and cheese.

Source: *Love and Lemons (loveandlemons.com)*

Sources of Alt Milk–Making Equipment

+ **Milkmade Non-dairy Milk Maker** by Chefe ($249.95) (mychef wave.com)
+ **Nutr Machine** ($169.00) (thenutr.com)
+ **The Big Cheese Making Kit:** Makes 20 batches of cheese for $26.73. The kit makes six types: mozzarella, ricotta, mascarpone, halloumi, feta, and parmesan. (bigcheesemakingkit.com)

Water and Other Beverages

Sources of Reverse Osmosis or Distillation Filters

+ **AquaTru** (aquatru.com; go to darinolien.com for a $100 discount)
+ **Vevor** (vevor.com)
+ **H2oLabs** (h2olabs.com)

Sources of Trace Minerals and Pink Himalayan Salt to Add to Distilled Water

+ **The Spice Lab** (for pink Himalayan salt) (spices.com)
+ **The Original Salt Company** (theoriginalsaltcompany.com)

+ **SaltWorks** (seasalt.com)
+ **Trace Mineral Drops** (concentrated complex of full-spectrum, naturally occurring ionic trace minerals from Utah's inland sea) (available at iherb.com)
+ **Quinton** (ocean minerals) (quicksilverscientific.com)

Sources of Healthy Canned and Bottled Beverages, Including Water

+ **Poppi** (drinkpoppi.com)
+ **Recess:** Sparkling water infused with hemp and adaptogens (takearecess.com)
+ **Olipop:** Gut-friendly soda (drinkolipop.com)
+ **PathWater:** Bottled in aluminum (not ideal but better than plastic); the company gives back to environmental/social justice causes (drinkpathwater.com)
+ **FreeWater:** An innovative advertising platform that utilizes spring water as a new medium while prioritizing philanthropy and sustainability (freewater.io)
+ **Mananalu:** Jason Momoa's aluminum bottled water company (mananalu.com)

Sources of Glass and Heavy Metal–Free Bottles

+ **Flaska:** Provides structured water from embedded frequencies in its glass bottles (flaska.us)
+ **Blue Bottle Love:** Frequency bottles; use promo code DARIN (bluebottlelove.com)
+ **The One Movement:** Sustainable bottles that combat plastic pollution in the ocean (theonemovement.co)
+ **Hydro Flask:** Certified lead-free bottles (hydroflask.com)
+ **Klean Kanteen:** Certified heavy metal–free bottles (kleankanteen.com)

Additional Resources

+ **Find a Spring:** Lists local spring water sources (findaspring.com)

Meat and Poultry

Black Bean Burger

Before you decide you need meat, try this DIY black bean burger.

1 flax "egg" (1 tablespoon flaxseed meal + 3 tablespoons water, beaten together)
1 teaspoon olive oil
1/2 red onion, finely diced
2–3 cloves garlic, minced
1 large carrot, shredded
1 (15 ounce) can black beans, rinsed and drained
1/4–1/3 cup oat flour, gluten free if desired
1 teaspoon cumin
1/2 teaspoon garlic powder
1 teaspoon chili powder
1/2 teaspoon paprika
1/2 teaspoon salt

Mix everything, form into patties, cook right away or store in the freezer.

Source: *CU Anschutz Health and Wellness Center (anschutzwellness.com)*

Eating a variety of plant-based protein, including grains, legumes, nuts, and seeds, can provide adequate amino acids and protein, just as animal flesh does. Here are some examples:

+ Tempeh: 16 grams of protein per cup
+ Edamame: 12 grams of protein per cup
+ Tofu: 11 grams of protein per cup
+ Soy milk: 4 grams of protein per cup

- Almond milk: 24 grams of protein per cup
- Hemp milk: 12 grams of protein per cup
- Barukas nuts: 6 grams of protein per cup
- Pistachio nuts: 6 grams of protein per cup
- Pumpkin seeds: 10 grams of protein per cup
- Quinoa: 4 grams of protein per cup
- Chickpea pasta: 13 grams of protein per cup
- Oats: 4 grams of protein per cup
- Brown rice: 3 grams of protein per cup
- Couscous: 3 grams of protein per cup
- Lentils: 9 grams of protein per 100 grams uncooked
- White beans: 9.7 grams of protein per 100 grams uncooked
- Split peas: 8.3 grams of protein per 100 grams uncooked
- Pinto beans: 9 grams of protein per 100 grams uncooked
- Kidney beans: 8.7 grams of protein per 100 grams uncooked
- Black beans: 8.9 grams of protein per 100 grams uncooked
- Navy beans: 8.2 grams of protein per 100 grams uncooked

You can always supplement your diet with a vegan protein powder of your choice!

Sources of Clean, Plant-Based Foods

- **Upton's Naturals** (uptonsnaturals.com)
- **Big Mountain Foods** (bigmountainfoods.com)
- **Better Nature** (betternaturetempeh.co)
- **The Jackfruit Company** (thejackfruitcompany.com)
- **Actual Veggies** (actualveggies.com)

If You Must Eat Meat, Try These Ethical, Sustainable, Organic Brands

- **Wild Pastures:** Grass fed, pasture raised; regenerative farming (wild pastures.com)

+ **Seven Sons:** Regenerative; pasture raised (sevensons.net)
+ **Cooks Venture:** Regenerative, organic, humane farming (cooks venture.com)
+ **U.S. Wellness Meats:** Sustainable land management; grass fed (grasslandbeef.com)

Additional Resources

Consult "Decoding Meat and Dairy Product Labels," on the EWG website, to research standards for meat and poultry. (ewg.org)

Fish Substitutes

DIY Vegan Tuna

1¹/₂ cups cooked chickpeas, or a 15.5-ounce can of chickpeas, drained (from non-BPA cans)
¹/₄ cup vegan mayonnaise
1 nori sheet, finely chopped
¹/₄ cup finely chopped red onion
1 tablespoon lemon juice
10 capers, finely chopped
¹/₂ teaspoon garlic powder
1 tablespoon nutritional yeast
1 tablespoon tamari or non-GMO soy sauce
¹/₂ tablespoon Dijon mustard
¹/₂ teaspoon white vinegar
Salt and pepper to taste

Place the chickpeas in a mixing bowl. Mash them with a fork. Mix with the other ingredients.

Source: *Loving It Vegan (lovingitvegan.com)*

Legumes are a great, protein-rich vegan fish substitute—try soybeans, black beans, chickpeas, white beans, yellow peas, green peas, black-eyed peas, and others.

Alternative Sources of Protein and Omega-3 Fatty Acids

+ **Brussels sprouts:** Each 1.5-ounce serving of cooked Brussels sprouts contains 44 milligrams of alpha-linoleic acid (ALA), 4 percent of the daily recommended intake.
+ **Algal oil:** Depending on the supplement, provides 400–500 milligrams of docosahexaenoic acid (DHA) and eicosapentaenoic acid (EPA), fulfilling 44–167 percent of the daily recommended intake. Recommended sources:
    ~ **Performance Lab:** Vegan, non-GMO, GMP certified, mercury free, and free from banned substances (performance lab.com)
    ~ **Vegetology:** Vegan, 100 percent lab grown (vegetology.com)
    ~ **Algamega:** Vegan, non-GMO, closed-system cultivation; contains both DHA and EPA (algamega.net)
+ **Chia seeds:** Best bought as whole seeds; grind with a coffee grinder or dry blender as needed.
+ **Flaxseeds:** Best bought as whole seeds; grind with a coffee grinder or dry blender as needed. Recommended products:
    ~ **Bob's Red Mill Flaxseed** (bobsredmill.com)
    ~ **Spectrum Essentials Organic Ground Premium Flaxseed** (spectrumorganics.com)
    ~ **Terrasoul Brown Flax Seeds** (terrasoul.com)
+ **Walnuts:** 1 ounce contains 2,570 milligrams of ALA omega-3 fatty acids, 160–233 percent of the daily recommended intake.
+ **Spirulina:** Contains omega-3 fatty acids in the form of ALA, EPA, and DHA. Recommended product:
    ~ **Raw Living Spirulina** (rawlivingspirulina.com)
+ **Tofu and tempeh:** Derived from soybeans, they contain 8 grams of protein per 100 grams.
+ **Quinoa:** 100 grams of quinoa contain 4 grams of protein. Quinoa contains all twenty-two amino acids.

Excellent options exist for those who crave seafood flavor without the harm involved. These are processed foods, of course, but they're okay to eat every once in a while.

Recommended Brands

+ **Good Catch** (goodcatchfoods.com)
+ **Gardein** (gardein.com)
+ **BeLeaf** (beleafvegan.com)
+ **Sophie's Kitchen** (sophieskitchen.com)
+ **The Plant-Based Food Seafood Co.** (plantbasedseafoodco.com)

Produce

DIY: grow your own, if you can. **Love the Garden** (lovethegarden.com) has great info on how to do it in easy, practical ways. If you have some land to work with, you can look into permaculture and/or regenerative agriculture at **Food Forest Abundance** (foodforestabundance.com).

The Environmental Working Group publishes a list of nonorganic produce you can safely buy, which it calls "The Clean 15":

+ Sweet corn (always choose non-GMO)
+ Onions
+ Cabbage
+ Asparagus
+ Avocados
+ Pineapples
+ Mangoes
+ Honeydew melon
+ Sweet peas
+ Papaya
+ Kiwi

+ Mushrooms
+ Cantaloupe
+ Sweet potatoes
+ Watermelon

Organic Produce

Organic food is 20 to 40 percent higher in antioxidants than nonorganic, and it doesn't have added antibiotics, hormones, or synthetic additives that can result in serious health complications.

Where to Find More Information

+ **USDA Organic Food Finder** (https://organic.ams.usda.gov/integrity) (USDA Organic Integrity Database)

Tips for Buying and Eating Organic Food on a Budget

+ Grow sprouts. To find out how, read *The Sprout Book: Tap into the Power of the Planet's Most Nutritious Food* by Doug Evans.
+ Shop at your local farmers' market.
+ Buy food in bulk.
+ Cook instead of ordering in or eating out.
+ Buy seasonal.
+ Buy frozen food instead of fresh (it's cheaper and may be more nutritious).
+ Keep in mind that proper storage extends foods' shelf life.
+ Buy only what you need.

Imperfect Foods (imperfectfoods.com) and **Misfits Market** (misfits market.com) have wonderful deals on produce and are an amazing way to cut down on waste and save money.

ELECTROMAGNETIC RADIATION

Wi-Fi

As I've already said, your safest bet is never to use wireless. Switch to using Ethernet whenever possible. Ethernet is faster than Wi-Fi, anyway! The fastest Ethernet speeds hit 10 gigabytes per second (Gbps) or higher, whereas Wi-Fi tops out at 6.9 Gbps. **Tech Wellness** (techwellness.com) is a great source of plug-in options.

If for some reason you cannot use Ethernet, find another way to minimize your exposure to router radiation.

+ Turn your router off at night and when you're not using it.
+ Stay as far away from your router as possible.

Products for Reducing EMF Exposure

EMF Meters

+ **Safe and Sound Pro II** (techwellness.com)
+ **Erickhill EMF Meter** (available at amazon.com)
+ **Latnex AF-5000 Multifield 5G EMF Meter** (available at emrss.com)
+ **TriField EMF Meter Model TF2** (emrss.com)

Remote Switches to Turn Off Routers

+ **Wi-Fi Switch Remote** (techwellness.com)

EMF-Blocking Clothing

+ **Conscious Spaces** (consciousspaces.com)
+ **Lambs:** Beanies, underwear, and hats that claim to block 99 percent of EMFs (getlambs.com)

USB to Ethernet Converters

Get one of these so you can connect your various devices to the Ethernet.

+ **Insignia** (insigniaproducts.com)
+ **Verrosa** (verrosa.com)

Sources of Router Shields

+ **Faraday Defense** (faradaydefense.com)
+ **EMF Essentials** (emfessentials.com)

Low-Radiation Routers

+ **JRS Eco 100 D1 on Asus:** Emits radiation only when Wi-Fi is being used (jrseco.com)
+ **Waveguard:** Minimizes EMF/5G/Wi-Fi radiation (waveguard .com/en)

Cell Phones

Sources of EMF-Blocking Phone Accessories

+ **SafeSleeve** (safesleevecases.com)
+ **Waveguard** (to carry with you or for room) (waveguard.com/en)
+ **SLNT** (slnt.com)

Source of Other Safe Electronic Accessories

+ **GoDark Bags** (godarkbags.com)

Headphones

If you use headphones, ditch the Bluetooth earbuds and get wired.

+ **EMF Protection Airtube Earphones** (techwellness.com)
+ **EMF Radiation-Free Earbuds Air Tube Stereo Headphones** (defendershield.com)

- **EMF Radiation-Free Air Tube Kids Headphones** (defender shield.com)
- **RF wireless headphones** (available at bestbuy.com and other stores)
- **Sennheiser RF headphones** (available at bestbuy.com and other stores)
- **Wired headphones** (available at walmart.com and other stores)

Airport Body Scanners

Instead of passing through the scanner, you have the legal right to opt out by allowing a TSA agent to pat you down. But allow some extra time for that to be done.

CLOTHING

Cotton and Denim

Shop secondhand. Not only is this a sustainable option, but used clothing generally contains fewer chemicals because it has been washed many times.

Sources of Secondhand Clothing

- **ThredUp** (thredup.com)
- **eBay** (ebay.com)
- **Mercari** (mercari.com)
- **Poshmark** (poshmark.com)
- **Depop** (depop.com)

Sources of Organic Fabric Clothing

- **Candiani Denim** (candianidenim.com)
- **Pact** (wearpact.com)
- **Everlane** (everlane.com)
- **Lucy & Yak** (lucyandyak.com)

+ **FatFace** (us.fatface.com)
+ **Nudie Jeans** (nudiejeans.com)
+ **Thought** (wearethought.com)
+ **Toad&Co** (toadandco.com)
+ **Patagonia** (patagonia.com)
+ **Quince** (onequince.com)
+ **Known Supply** (knownsupply.com)
+ **Tentree** (tentree.com)
+ **Crann Organic** (crannorganic.com)

Sources of Sustainable, Healthy Cotton T-Shirts

+ **Certton** (certton.com.au)
+ **Blessed Earth** (blessedearth.com.au)
+ **Organic Embrace** (organicembrace.com.au)
+ **Organic Basics** (us.organicbasics.com)
+ **Brook There** (brookthere.com)
+ **Thought** (wearethought.com)

Waterproof Clothing

Use a safe, nontoxic spray or wax to waterproof your clothing at home, for example:

+ **Nikwax PFA-Free Clothing Waterproof Wax** (rei.com)
+ **DetraPel PFA Waterproof Clothing Spray** (detrapel.com)

Sources of Nontoxic Waterproof Clothing and Gear

+ **Icebreaker** (icebreaker.com)
+ **Nau** (nau.com)
+ **prAna** (prana.com)
+ **Houdini Sportswear** (houdinisportswear.com)
+ **Páramo** (paramo-clothing.com)
+ **Didriksons** (didriksons.com)

+ **Picture Organic Clothing** (picture-organic-clothing.com/en)
+ **Deuter** (deuter.com)
+ **Royal Robbins** (royalrobbins.com)
+ **TheTentLab** (thetentlab.com)

Vegan Leather

Vegan Leather Coats

+ **Bernardo Neo Active Double Up Hooded Puffer** (bernardo fashions.com)
+ **Noize Women's GIGI Heavyweight Parka** (noize.com)
+ **Save the Duck USA Women's Colette Long Puffer Coat** (savethe duckusa.com)
+ **Save the Duck USA Men's Alter Hooded Parka** (savetheduck usa.com)
+ **Harper Coats The Brunch Puffer** (harpercoats.com)
+ **Matt & Nat** (mattandnat.com)

Sources of Vegan Leather Handbags

+ **Pixie Mood:** This company has introduced cork into its products, started using expanded polyethylene (EPE) foam packaging, and uses recycled vegan leather. Its collections include tote bags, shoulder bags, cross-body bags, and bucket bags. (pixiemood.com)
+ **Gunas USA:** Uses PETA-approved vegan leather (gunasthe brand.com)
+ **Watson & Wolfe:** This company specializes in vegan wallets and eco-friendly accessories. It also sells handbags. (watsonwolfe.com)
+ **Melie Bianco:** 100 percent vegan and sweatshop-free bags (melie bianco.com)
+ **Doshi:** Smart, fashionable, high-quality vegan bags, belts, wallets, backpacks, briefcases, and more. It uses recyclable, biodegradable, durable, and sustainable materials. (doshi.shop)

Vegan Shoe Brands

+ **Aera** (aeranewyork.com)
+ **Avesu Vegan Shoes** (avesuveganshoes.com)
+ **Bhava** (bhavastudio.com)
+ **Blue District** (shopbluedistrict.com)
+ **Brave Gentleman** (bravegentleman.com)
+ **Indosole** (indosole.com)
+ **MooShoes** (mooshoes.com)
+ **Sylth Virago** (sylthvirago.com)
+ **Taylor + Thomas** (taylorandthomasla.com)
+ **Vivobarefoot** (vivobarefoot.com)

Vegan/Sustainable Clothing

+ **Amur:** Makes fashionable women's wear from recycled materials, organic cotton, and cellulose (amur.com)
+ **Ccilu:** Uses innovative technology to create eco-friendly shoes, recycling commonly discarded materials such as coffee grounds and plastic bottles (ccilu.com)
+ **Brave Gentleman:** Uses materials such as recycled soda and water bottles, as well as recycled polyester/cotton blends diverted from waste streams (bravegentleman.com)
+ **Reformation:** On-trend designs and high-quality fabrics, made partially from recycled vintage clothing (thereformation.com)
+ **Loomstate:** Vegan-friendly brand that's committed to using 100 percent certified organic cotton in its designs in order to keep the environment clean and farmers healthy (loomstate.org)
+ **Parley for the Oceans:** Is trying to clean all the world's seas of plastic debris and pollution. Part of the effort involves fashion collaborations with Adidas, fabric makers, even artists creating bags, sunglasses, and other products. (parley.tv)

+ **Patagonia:** Has been recycling plastic bottles for use in its outerwear and other clothing since the 1990s. It takes plastic from the ocean and recycles that, too. (patagonia.com)
+ **Wuxly:** Local production that limits its carbon footprint. It is committed to reducing CO_2 emissions and further supports efforts to protect wildlife. (wuxly.com)

Underwear

+ **Wolf x Rose:** My favorite! Healthy, clean, organic cotton garments by my good buddy and designer Jeff Garner. (wolfxrose.com)
+ **WAMA Underwear:** The company estimates that it's saved 283,277 days' worth of drinking water and 297,560 hours' worth of LED bulb energy. (wamaunderwear.com)
+ **Knickey:** Certified as climate neutral, it uses responsibly produced organic cotton, ensures fair labor standards from manufacturers, and has an underwear recycling program. Also, it releases a detailed impact report that covers sustainability improvements each year. (knickey.com)
+ **TomboyX:** Sizes that range from 3XS to 6X and nongendered styles. TomboyX is B Corp certified, meaning that it meets B Lab's rigorous standards for social and environmental impact as well as continued accountability and transparency about its practices. Though it does not use organic cotton, the fabric has been tested for harmful materials. (tomboyx.com)
+ **Arq:** Products come from a family-owned sewing factory that uses sustainably dyed fabrics. (shoparq.com)
+ **Oddobody:** Materials are completely compostable. Furthermore, the company uses a family-run manufacturer in Peru and regularly visits the factories and farms that create the underwear. (oddo body.com)

Organic Cotton Underwear Brands

+ **Pact:** Cotton basics for every gender and size (wearpact.com)
+ **Boody:** Collections made from sustainably grown bamboo viscose (boody.com)
+ **Brook There:** Sustainable lingerie made from organic cotton and natural silk (brookthere.com)
+ **Proclaim:** Wide range of products made from Tencel or Repreve, a polyester fiber made from recycled plastic water bottles (wearproclaim.com)
+ **Huha:** Produced with a natural antibacterial that looks to keep your "huha" healthy. The company uses Tencel as its main material and ships plastic free. (hu-ha.com)
+ **Cosabella:** Luxury lingerie made in Italy since 1983. Handmade in family-run workshops. (cosabella.com)
+ **Cuup:** Bra sizes ranging from A to H, sustainable materials and ethical practices (shopcuup.com)
+ **Girlfriend Collective:** Bras and undies made with recycled plastic from water bottles. They can be recycled again through its ReGirlfriend initiative when you no longer need it. (girlfriend.com)
+ **Organic Basics:** Bra sizes from 30A to 38C and XS to XL. The enterprise focuses on sustainable materials such as regenerative organic cotton and Tencel and ethical production. (organicbasics.com)
+ **Tentree:** Made with Tencel, organic cotton, and Refibra lyocell, in which upcycled cotton scraps are turned into cotton pulp and then combined with wood pulp. Even the elastic trims are made using recycled materials. Plus, it is certified B Corp, and for every purchase, the company plants ten trees. (tentree.com)

Tights

+ **Swedish Stockings:** Sustainable hosiery with a vast range of colors and styles of recycled tights. (swedishstockings.com)

+ **Kintra:** An emerging company that is eliminating petroleum in the development of textiles. Derived from sugar monomers that decompose after use. (kintrafibers.com)
+ **Dear Denier:** Tights made from recycled polyamide and elastane with low-waste production practices. Plus, the company has a water recycling management system and offers a recycling program that accepts tights from any brand. (deardenier.com)

Fabric Dyes

+ **Earth Pigments** (earthpigments.com)
+ **Organic Cotton Plus** (organiccottonplus.com)
+ **NatureColorsEU** (available at etsy.com)
+ **Jacquard** (available at amazon.com)
+ **Cutch Natural Dye** (available at etsy.com)

DIY Organic Tie-Dye Process

White cotton fabric for dyeing
Rubber bands
Gloves
Vinegar or salt (as a fixative)
Water
Various pots and pans
Containers for dyeing
Small strainer
Raw materials to make dyes; for example, turmeric powder
    for yellow; red onion skins for pink; red cabbage leaves for
    purple

Prepare the fabric for dyeing. Use the rubber bands to create a pattern on the fabric. Once you're satisfied with your design, it's time to treat your fabric with a fixative. If you are making a berry-based dye, mix 1/2 cup of salt with 8 cups of water and bring to a boil. Simmer your fabric in the solution for one hour prior to dyeing. If you are making a plant/veggie-based dye, mix 1 part vinegar to 4 parts water and follow the same process. When done simmering, run the fabric under cool water and wring out a bit of the excess water.

Make the dye. Wearing gloves, cut or tear the raw ingredients into small pieces and measure. Place into a pot and pour in water (2 parts water to 1 part raw ingredients; for example, 1 cup of torn cabbage leaves to 2 cups of water). If you are using a spice such as turmeric, the proportions will be 1–2 tablespoons of spice to 3–4 cups of water. Bring the mixture to a boil and simmer for about an hour. The longer you cook it, the more intense your color will become. When done simmering, strain dye into a container or jar big enough to fit your garment or fabric. You will feel a bit like a mad scientist at this point, but just go with it!

Dye the fabric. Wearing gloves, place the fabric into the dye containers and allow it to rest for a while. We didn't play around with using multiple colors on a single garment, but you could experiment with placing dye in a bottle with an applicator and squirting it directly onto the fabric, as many people do when tie-dyeing. Once the fabric has reached the desired hue (the color will lighten a little as your fabric dries), remove it from the dye and rinse with cool water until the water runs clear. Remove the rubber bands and hang the clothing to dry.

Source: *Grove Collaborative (grove.com)*

OEKO-TEX Certification

OEKO-TEX has several labels that identify whether textiles from towels to clothing have been tested for harmful substances. Its Standard 100 label uses the European Chemical Agency's list of substances of very high concern and other regulations to determine if any harmful substances were used in manufacturing, while the Made in Green label also ensures sustainable manufacturing. You can also enter a product's OEKO-TEX label number into OEKO-TEX's Label Check and trace the product back to its production facility. (oeko-tex.com/en/label-check)

HOUSEHOLD PRODUCTS

Cookware

+ **Anodized aluminum** is treated with an acidic solution that changes how the metal behaves. It is easier to clean and can have nonstick qualities. Plus, it supposedly doesn't cause leaching of aluminum into your food to the extent that regular aluminum does.
+ **Stainless steel** is an alloy that typically contains iron, chrome, and nickel. Resistant to rust and corrosion, it distributes heat evenly over its surface. As long as you grease or oil the pan before cooking and soak it in water right afterward, it's easy to clean. There's little reason to believe that cooking with stainless steel is harmful, but it may aggravate a sensitivity or allergy to nickel.
+ **Ceramic cookware** is most likely safe, but not enough research has been done to be sure. Always read the label, as some brands may include Teflon.

Sources of Safe Cookware

+ **Rad USA:** Anodized aluminum, nonstick cookware by my good buddy, chef Oren Zroya (radusa.co)
+ **Caraway:** Teflon, PFAS, and heavy metal free (carawayhome.com)
+ **360 Cookware:** Nontoxic stainless-steel cookware options (360cookware.com)
+ **Milo Cookware:** This brand focuses on longevity, sustainability, and conscious production. Its cookware is crafted from 40 percent nonstick recycled cast iron sprayed with TOMATEC enamel. (available at kanalifestyle.com)
+ **Made In:** Artisan-made, nonstick, nontoxic stainless-steel cookware (oven safe up to 800°F) and carbon-steel cookware (oven safe up to 1,200°F) (madeincookware.com)
+ **Smithey Ironware:** Heirloom-quality hand-forged carbon-steel and cast-iron cookware (smithey.com)

+ **Great Jones:** Stainless-steel pots and pans, ceramic nonstick cookware sets, and cast-iron skillets that are oven safe and display worthy. Free from PFOA and PTFE chemicals. (greatjonesgoods.com)

Safety Tips

+ Unless you're using glass or stone bakeware, don't store food in the pot or pan it was cooked in.
+ Avoid cleaning cookware with rough materials or metal mesh, which can scratch and compromise surfaces.
+ Minimize the amount of time your food is in contact with metals from pots and pans.
+ Use as little olive oil, coconut oil, or cooking spray as possible to minimize the amount of cookware coating that sticks to your food.
+ Clean pots and pans thoroughly after each use.
+ Replace cookware every two to three years or as soon as you notice any gouges or scratches in the coating.

Aluminum Foil

Avoid aluminum altogether! That should be easy to remember. Exposure can result in respiratory and neurological problems. It has even been linked to Alzheimer's disease. Also, it is not environmentally friendly. However, if you feel you must use it, anodized aluminum is the safest option.

Anodized Aluminum Brands

+ **Ninja Foodi NeverStick:** PTFE nonstick coat that's PFOA free (ninjakitchen.com)
+ **T-fal Ultimate:** Nonstick and PFOA free (available in stores such as Kohl's and Bed Bath & Beyond)
+ **Calphalon:** Three layers of PFOA-free nonstick coating (available at amazon.com)

- **Cuisinart Chef's Classic:** Has a hard anodized coating that is PFOA-free, scratch resistant, and durable (cuisinart.com)
- **Rachael Ray:** Has a PTFE nonstick coat that's PFOA free (available at wayfair.com)
- **Cook N Home:** Is PFOA free (available at wayfair.com)

Safe Food Wraps

- **Earth Hero reusable food wraps** (earthhero.com)
- **Cedar food wraps** (available at amazon.com)
- **LilyBee wraps** (lilybeewrap.com)
- **Silicon reusable sandwich wraps** (available at amazon.com)
- **Nordic by Nature reusable sandwich bags** (nordicbynature bags.com)
- **Khala & Co. Reusable Vegan Food Wraps** (available at earth hero.com)
- **Responsible Products Certified Compostable Food Bags** (responsibleproducts.com)

Plastic Food Containers

Don't use them! Glass, ceramic, metal, wood, and bamboo are all safe alternatives. If you must use plastic:

- Never microwave food in anything other than ceramic or glass.
- Don't put them into the dishwasher; don't allow plastic to get that hot.
- Check the recycling code on the bottom of containers, and avoid plastics with recycling codes 3, 6, and 7, which may contain phthalates, styrene, and bisphenols, unless they are labeled "biobased" or "greenware," indicating that they're made from corn.

Safe Storage Containers

Stainless Steel

- **Thrive Market** (thrivemarket.com)
- **Package Free** (packagefreeshop.com)
- **Thanos** (available at wayfair.com)
- **Bentgo** (bentgo.com)
- **Rebrilliant food storage containers** (available at wayfair.com)
- **Life Without Plastic** (lifewithoutplastic.com)

Glass

- **Crate & Barrel** (crateandbarrel.com)
- **Package Free** (packagefreeshop.com)
- **Ikea** (ikea.com)
- **DE plastic-free glass food storage containers** (available at amazon.com)

Ceramic

- **CorningWare French White 24-Inch Baking Dish with Lid** (corningware.com)
- **Marie Kondo Cloud White Modular Ceramic Canisters** (available at containerstore.com)

Cloth Bags (for Dry Foods)

- **Veggie Saver** (veggiesaver.com)

Another way to go plastic free is to buy products from **Shopetee** (shopetee.com), an online store for containers as well as toothbrushes and more.

Sheets, Bedding, and Pillows

Sources

+ **Parachute Home:** Climate Neutral certified, Global Organic Textile Standard (GOTS) certified, and OEKO-TEX certified. Timeless and durable essentials with various organic options. (parachute home.com)
+ **Ettitude:** Uses CleanBamboo, which is sourced from FSC-certified sustainable forests and made in a nontoxic, closed-loop system that recycles 98 percent of water (ettitude.com)
+ **HauteCoton:** From seed to consumer. All products are thoughtfully crafted and responsibly sourced at every stage of production. (haute coton.com)
+ **Eucalypso Home:** Sheets with 100 percent Tencel lyocell from natural eucalyptus fibers, which are cultivated using one-tenth the amount of water used to cultivate cotton and are milled in a zero-footprint, OEKO-TEX-certified environment in Austria. (eucalypso home.com)
+ **Coyuchi:** Uses a high proportion of eco-friendly materials, including GOTS cotton (coyuchi.com)
+ **Buffy:** Known for sustainably manufacturing products using fibers made from eucalyptus, hemp, and recycled plastic (buffy.co)

Sources of Organic Bedding

+ **The Beach People:** Infuses eucalyptus fiber, a hypoallergenic, breathable, long-lasting material, into its fabric blends to create a silk-like material (thebeachpeople.co)
+ **Mulberry Threads:** Makes organic bamboo bedsheets (mulberry threads.com)
+ **Made Trade:** Stocks organic sheets, sustainable robes, and ethically made towels from brands such as Area Home and Hoot's (made trade.com)

+ **West Elm:** Stocks products made from linen, organic cotton, and a variety of other luxurious fabrics (westelm.com)
+ **Bhumi Organic Cotton:** Uses organic cotton to completely eliminate the harmful effects of conventional cotton on farmers, their families, and surrounding villages (bhumiorganic.com)
+ **Under the Canopy:** Bedding, bath, and apparel (underthecanopy.com)

Furniture and Upholstery

Sources of Nontoxic Products

+ **Savvy Rest:** Made from organic fabrics such as cotton, hemp, and wool; natural Talalay latex foam; solid wood; and more. The company has various third-party certifications for sustainability and safety, including GOTS, Cradle to Cradle, and GREENGUARD. Free from PFAS, flame retardants, formaldehyde glue, cardboard, metal coils, particleboard, plywood, and veneer. (savvyrest.com)
+ **Burrow:** Nontoxic, free from PFASs and flame retardants. CertiPUR-US certified. (burrow.com)
+ **Carolina Morning:** Beds made from locally harvested Appalachian poplar wood and finished with a nontoxic finish and cushions made with 100 percent certified organic cotton canvas, then filled with natural and eco-friendly kapok fiber. (zafu.net)
+ **Medley:** Uses FSC-certified solid wood for its frames with zero-VOC glues. In its foam cushions you can choose between CertiPUR-US-certified foam and certified organic natural Dunlop latex. All free from flame retardants. (medleyhome.com)
+ **Sabai:** Free from formaldehyde, flame retardants, and PFASs. Their cushions are made from CertiPUR-US foam, their fabrics are untreated, and the wood used for the frames is FSC certified and finished with a low-VOC stain. (sabai.design)
+ **Natural Home:** Fabric options include organic cotton, linen, and wool. Free from PFASs. (thefutonshop.com)

+ **Ecobalanza:** Uses nontoxic zero-VOC glues and Rubio Monocoat stains (ecobalanza.com)
+ **Pure Upholstery:** Organic latex with a feather and down wrap, solid maple wood, organic wool, GOTS-certified organic cotton, PFAS free, GREENGUARD-certified water-based glue, and Rubio Monocoat wood finish on legs. No flame retardants. (pure upholstery.com)
+ **Cisco Home:** Inside Green option contains organic natural latex wrapped in either eco-wool or feathers and down. The company uses certified solid woods, organic cotton fabrics with no toxic treatments, jute and hemp instead of springs, and WOCA natural stains. Free from flame retardants. (ciscohome.net)

Carpeting

In General

+ Choose solid wood flooring with a low-VOC finish.
+ Choose tile with a low-VOC sealant.
+ Choose cork or natural linoleum when possible.

What to Look For in a Carpet

+ Nontreated fibers
+ Zero VOC (ideal)
+ Made of wool or cotton
+ Padding made from wool or felt
+ Green Label Plus or GREENGUARD low-VOC certification
+ No stain or waterproofing treatments
+ Low-VOC adhesives or fastener system
+ Handmade
+ Ethically and sustainably produced

Sources of Good-Quality Rugs

+ **Revival:** Organic cotton, wool, hemp, and other healthy materials (revivalrugs.com)
+ **Nestig:** Organic cotton and nontoxic dyes (nestig.com)
+ **The Citizenry:** Ethically and sustainably made; nontoxic (the -citizenry.com)
+ **Lorena Canals:** Handmade by artists in northern India, using only recycled and natural fibers (such as cotton and wool) and nontoxic dyes. They are machine washable. (lorenacanals.us)
+ **West Elm:** Nontoxic; made from jute, hemp, seagrass, and other healthy materials (westelm.com)
+ **Ruggable:** Machine washable; water-based dyes; no harsh chemicals. The company donates part of its proceeds to One Tree Planted, Best Friends Animal Society, and Baby2Baby. (ruggable.com)

Air-Conditioning

Sources of Air Conditioners

+ **Evapolar:** Eco friendly, using no freonlike liquids. Energy and cost efficient, too. (evapolar.com)
+ **EcoCooling:** Natural, cost efficient, and environmentally friendly. (ecocooling.co.uk)
+ **Hessaire:** Cost efficient and eco friendly. (hessaire.com)

Sources of Whole-House Fans

+ **QuietCool** (quietcoolsystems.com)
+ **Whole House Fan** (wholehousefan.com)
+ **Cool Attic** (available at amazon.com)

Sources of Ductless Mini-split Air Conditioners

+ **Senville** (senville.com)
+ **Cooper & Hunter** (available on cooperandhunter.us)
+ **Pioneer** (pioneerminisplit.com)

Air Fresheners

DIY Air Freshener No. 1

Fill a glass spray bottle halfway with witch hazel. Fill rest of the bottle with distilled water. Add 25–30 drops of essential oils (not fragrance oils). Add dried flowers (optional). Shake and spray.

Source: *Martha Stewart (marthastewart.com)*

DIY Air Freshener No. 2

10 drops lavender essential oil
10 drops vanilla essential oil
1 tablespoon witch hazel
Any other essential oil of your choice

Combine all ingredients in a glass spray bottle.

Source: *Joy Food Sunshine (diynatural.com)*

Air Purifiers

+ **Therapure** (envion.com)
+ **Coway Airmega Mighty** (available at amazon.com)
+ **Coway Airmega 200M** (available at walmart.com)
+ **Levoit Core 300** (available at homedepot.com)
+ **Medify Air MA-14** (available at amazon.com)

Essential Oil Diffusers

+ **Grove Co. Essential Oil Burner** (grove.co)
+ **Aroma Om Deluxe Diffuser** (available at saje.com)
+ **TerraFuse Deluxe Diffuser** (available at planttherapy.com)

Microwave Ovens

If you are at home, use a regular stove or oven instead of a microwave. Even if it might take longer, it is better for you. Cooking can even have positive benefits to your mental health. If your home oven has a broiler option, this is another way to reheat your food and add a crispy texture.

Instant Pots and Pressure Cookers

+ **Ninja** (ninjakitchen.com)
+ **Instant Pot** (instantpot.com)
+ **T-fal USA** (t-falusa.com)
+ **Breville** (breville.com)

Toaster Ovens

+ **Hamilton Beach** (hamiltonbeach.com)
+ **KitchenAid** (kitchenaid.com)

Portable Food Warmers and Crockpots

+ **Crockpot** (crock-pot.com)
+ **Aotto** (aotto.com)
+ **Travelisimo** (travelisimobrand.com)

Laundry Detergent

DIY Laundry Detergent No. 1

1 5-ounce bar pure Castile soap
1 cup washing soda
1 cup baking soda
1 cup coarse salt

Place the Castile soap in the bowl of a food processor and blitz it until it's finely ground. If you don't have a food processor, finely chop the soap or use a cheese grater instead. The finer you can get it, the better.

Then, add your washing soda, baking soda, and salt. Blend until you have a fine powder.

Once it's well blended, store in a labeled glass jar with an airtight lid.

Use 2 tablespoons per load of laundry if you have a standard machine, and 1 tablespoon per load if you have a high-efficiency machine.

Source: *MindBodyGreen (mindbodygreen.com)*

DIY Laundry Detergent No. 2

$1/2$ cup Epsom salts
$1^1/2$ cups baking soda
$1^1/2$ cups washing soda
$1/4$ cup sea salt
20–25 drops essential oils of your choice

Mix all ingredients well, making sure to incorporate essential oils, if using, and blend in any clumps.

Store in glass jar of choice with a lid.

Use 1 heaping tablespoon per load (2 for extra soiled or extremely large loads).

Source: *Fresh Mommy Blog (freshmommyblog.com)*

Laundry Detergent Sheets

Most laundry detergent sheets are cost effective, great for the environment, and free from harsh chemicals and fragrances. Always make sure to get the unscented versions.

- **Tru Earth Eco-Strips Laundry Detergent** (tru.earth)
- **Earth Breeze Eco Sheets** (earthbreeze.com)
- **Sheets Laundry Club Laundry Detergent Sheets** (sheetslaundry club.com)
- **EcoRoots Laundry Detergent Sheets** (ecoroots.us)

Laundry Detergents

- **Branch Basics The Concentrate** (branchbasics.com)
- **Nature First Soap Berry Laundry Detergent Pods** (putnature first.com)
- **Simply Co. Laundry Detergent** (available at packagefreeshop.com)
- **Sea Salt Zum Laundry Soap** (indigowild.com)

All-Purpose Cleaning Products

For the following recipes, use distilled water, as tap water can cause streaking.

DIY Glass Cleaner No. 1

2 cups distilled water
1/2 cup white or apple cider vinegar

¼ cup rubbing alcohol 70 percent concentration
1–2 drops orange essential oil for scent (optional)

Combine the ingredients in a spray bottle.

Source: *Good Housekeeping (goodhouskeeping.com)*

DIY Glass Cleaner No. 2

One part white vinegar
One part distilled water

Combine the ingredients in a spray bottle. If you don't like the smell of vinegar (which dissipates quickly), you can add about 10 drops of your favorite essential oil and shake to mix.

Source: *The Spruce (thespruce.com)*

DIY All-Purpose Cleaner

One part white vinegar
One part water
¼ teaspoon grated lemon rind
Rosemary sprigs

Combine the ingredients in a spray bottle. Let infuse for one week before using.

Source: *The Spruce (thespruce.com)*

DIY Disinfectant Spray

2 cups distilled water
1 tablespoon white vinegar
A few drops of tea tree oil

Combine the ingredients in a spray bottle. If you like, add a couple drops of lavender or other essential oil for scent.

DIY Natural Heavy-Duty Scrub

1/2 lemon
1/2 cup borax powder

To remove rust stains on porcelain or enamel sinks and tubs, dip the cut side of the lemon into the borax and scrub the sink or tub's surface, then rinse. This is *not* safe for marble or granite. You can find borax, a laundry booster, in the supermarket detergent aisle or order it on Amazon.

Source: *Good Housekeeping (goodhouskeeping.com)*

Certifications and More Information

For more information on safe cleaning products, consult the following.

- **EPA Safer Choice:** Products with an EPA Safer Choice label not only contain ingredients that have been thoroughly researched and approved by the EPA but have also been tested for performance and sustainable packaging.
- **Environmental Working Group Guide to Healthy Cleaning:** A database for cleaning products. Because these products aren't required to disclose all ingredients, EWG researches "beyond the labels" to ensure that they are safe to use. (ewg.org/guides/cleaners)
- **EWG Verified:** If you prefer not to have to sift through the Healthy Cleaning database, an easy shortcut is to look for products that have the label EWG Verified. This label means that the product meets EWG's "strict, scientific standards for transparency and health," meaning that it doesn't contain any ingredients with health, ecotoxicity, or contamination concerns and that the manufacturer is transparent about all ingredients on its labels, including fragrance, and follows good manufacturing practices. Look for the EWG Verified seal on product labels.

+ **ECOLOGO:** UL Solutions certifies cleaning products with its ECOLOGO label that have a lower environmental impact in the manufacturing process. You can shop for these products on Amazon by searching for ECOLOGO.
+ **MADE SAFE:** The nonprofit Nontoxic Certified created the MADE SAFE seal to verify that household cleaning products are created with nontoxic ingredients and don't contain any of the 6,500 substances on its banned list. It also looks for products that are not going to persist and pollute our water, air, or soil. You can find products on its database, look for the MADE SAFE seal on their labels, or search for them on Amazon.

Suppliers of Safe Cleaning Products

+ **Seventh Generation** (seventhgeneration.com)
+ **Guests on Earth** (guestsonearth.com)
+ **Dr. Bronner's:** Its biodegradable cleaner is not organic but has an A rating from the EWG (drbronner.com)
+ **Grove Collaborative** (grove.co)
+ **Tru Earth** (tru.earth)
+ **The Honest Company** (honest.com)
+ **Koala Eco** (koalaeco.com)
+ **Greenshield Organic** (greenshieldorganic.com)
+ **Common Good** (commongoodandco.com)
+ **Better Life Unscented Glass Cleaner** (available at hivebrands.com)
+ **Meliora Cleaning Products** (meliorameansbetter.com)

ACKNOWLEDGMENTS

THIS BOOK WAS MORE CHALLENGING TO write than I imagined it would be. Nothing is clearer to me now: it takes a village to write a book. This one, at least.

What you see in these pages was maybe one-tenth of the research we had to find, go through, vet, and understand before we could put it all together.

I am extremely grateful to the village that got this book done.

I want to thank a force of nature named Karen Rinaldi and the entire team at Harper Wave for believing that I could push the envelope on this book.

I owe huge thanks and massive gratitude to my main partner/writer/editor, Bill Tonelli. We did my previous book, *SuperLife*, together, and this one was ten times as challenging. Bill showed grit, persistence, and professionalism. Without him this book would simply not be here. Bill, you rock. Thank you.

To my great book agent, Richard Pine, for being there, grounded and wise, and Eliza Rothstein and the whole team at InkWell Management.

To my whole team, which had to navigate me through more than a year of working on this book: my assistants Kirsten Asher and Indira Dejtia, and Melissa Maulin Fuir, Kaili Bonnyman, Corrine Cassels, Ronald Fernandes, and Thiago Veiga.

A huge thanks to Dr. Leonardo Trasande for becoming a new friend as well as educating me on endocrine disruptors in his great, thorough book *Sicker, Fatter, Poorer: The Urgent Threat of Hormone-Disrupting Chemicals to Our Health and Future . . . and What We Can Do About It.* I'm also grateful to Dr. Shanna H. Swan for her wise words about the dangers of endocrine disruptors and other chemicals we unknowingly take in. She's one of the world's leading environmental and reproductive epidemiologists and the author of *Count Down: How Our Modern World Is Threatening Sperm Counts, Altering Male and Female Reproductive Development, and Imperiling the Future of the Human Race.*

Massive gratitude goes to my good friend Paul Hawken and his life-long work with all his books as well as Regeneration (and his team) as he paves the road for people like me to try to build upon.

Special thanks to Raven Devanney for kicking ass and finding the researchers, organizing them, coordinating with them, and surviving the crazy path through the journey of this book.

And to all the researchers, the undergrads, master's and PhD student interns, the professionals, and the amateurs whom we were able to teach to be great, you all helped with the everything that went into this book. Thanks for hanging in there as we figured it out. Some of you lasted longer than others, but to all of you I am grateful.

And to the badasses who were with us the whole way!

Krissy Walter Lieser
Nathan Olien
Morgan Webb
Sydney Webb
Luz Verónica
Rebecca Harris
Heidi Hahn
Rachel Misch
Sally Richardson
Tammy See
Isabella Marzano

To the rest of you, thanks for all your hard work.

Jacob Kummerling
Suzan Chong
Renee Santangelo
Ryan Bradly
Alan Carr
Ashley Forest
Martha Elizabeth Baker
David Conner
Rebecca De Cosmis
Christina Laughlin
Cassidy Chalhoub
John Massart
Colin T

And finally, to the other professional editors and researchers who helped me with their expertise and ability to keep me from going completely, overwhelmingly mad: thank you, Sara Vigneri, John Jusino, and Ambrose Martos.

A NOTE ON SOURCES

FOR CITATIONS OF THE STUDIES AND articles we used in researching this book, go to https://darinolien.com/fatal-conveniences-book/. We have tried our best to be accurate, but please keep in mind that scientists are constantly learning new things and changing their minds, as they should.

INDEX

ABOUT THE AUTHOR

DARIN OLIEN is the cohost of the Emmy Award–winning Netflix docu-series *Down to Earth with Zac Efron*. He has spent nearly twenty years exploring the planet, discovering new and underutilized exotic foods and medicinal plants as a superfood hunter. Darin developed Shakeology for Beachbody and is the author of the *New York Times* bestselling book *SuperLife: The 5 Simple Fixes That Will Make You Healthy, Fit, and Eternally Awesome*. As the host of the widely popular podcast *The Darin Olien Show*, Darin explores people, solutions, and health as well as life's Fatal Conveniences. He is the founder of Barùkas—the most nutrient-dense nut in the world, from the Cerrado Savannah of Brazil. Darin holds a bachelor of arts in exercise physiology and nutrition and a master's in psychology.